Our correct web address and e-mail:
Web: cancersos.com
e-mail: cancrsos@iag.net
(errors on order forms in back of book)

CANCER S.O.S.

Strategies Of Survival

A GUIDEBOOK FOR WOMEN WITH CANCER

by

Rose Welsh and Shirley Grandahl

with Foreword by Jerome L. Belinson, M.D.

ALBA PUBLISHING, INC.

ALBA PUBLISHING, INC.

342 Alba Lane, Lake Mary, Florida 32746

First Published 1998

First Edition

© Rose Welsh and Shirley Grandahl

Cover Design & Interior Illustration by Pamela S. Ross
Book Design & Typeset by Ross Studio Incorporated
Printed in Florida, U.S.A.
Set in Palatino Regular 10 pt.

Library of Congress Cataloguing
Rose Welsh, Shirley Grandahl
Cancer S.O.S., Strategies of Survival
LC# 97-94396
ISBN # 0-9660057-5-9

Warning/Disclaimer

This book is sold with the understanding that the publisher and authors are not engaged in rendering medical, legal, accounting, spiritual, mental or other professional services. If expert help is needed, the services of a competent professional should be engaged.

This book was not designed to provide all pertinent information on the subject of cancer, but to act as an aid and a complement to existing information. The publisher and authors suggest that you read all available information suitable to your situation and use this book as a supplement.

Every effort has been made by the publisher and authors to make this book as accurate and complete as possible. No warrants are made to accuracy of content or layout and design or for errors and omissions. The information in this book is dated as of publication date.

The purpose of this book is to assist the cancer patient. The publisher and authors have no liability or responsibility to any person or entity regarding damage or loss from information contained in this book either directly or indirectly.

You may not wish to be bound by the above and may return this book to the publisher for a full refund.

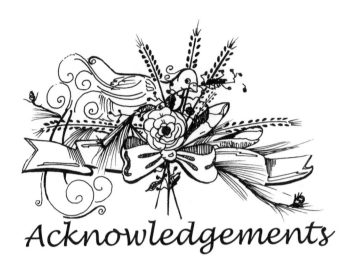

Acknowledgements

We are grateful to the following people for the contributions they made, in various ways, to the writing of this book: Our thanks to Dr. Jerome L. Belinson, Patricia Van Bramer, Dr. Susan Curry, Susan Drangenis, Judy Foster, P.A., R.N., Gary Gates, Jim Grandahl, Russ Grandahl, Linda House, R.N., Jan Jacobs, R.N., Barb Kulp, R.N., O.C.N., Greg Laurence, Jill Lee, Laurie Mingarelli, Bobbie Namm, R.N., Gurt Peterson R.N., O.C.N., Diane Pomeroy, Barbara Spadafora, Pamela Susan and Gregory Ross, Harry Rozelle, Susan Wallace, Vince Welsh and Rena Miller, and Falco Witkamp.

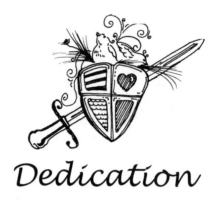

Dedication

To Russ and Gary who suffered and rejoiced with us.

Table of Contents

Introduction   Strategies of Survival... vii

Foreword   Walking In The Same Shoes..................................... 1

Chapter 1   STRATEGY #1: Understanding Your Diagnosis............   3
Chapter 2   STRATEGY #2: Getting All The Facts...........................   29
Chapter 3   STRATEGY #3: Taking Command....................................   43
Chapter 4   STRATEGY #4: Protecting Your Body From Infection...   75
Chapter 5   STRATEGY #5: Keeping a Positive Image.....................   91
Chapter 6   STRATEGY #6: Maintaining Control of Your Mind &
                            Body Through Nutrition & Exercise.... 103
Chapter 7   STRATEGY #7: Keeping Financial, Insurance & Legal
                            Concerns In Check................................ 123

Conclusion... 137
Appendix.. 138
Cancer Centers.. 148
Glossary... 151
Suggested Reading... 164
Bibliography... 165
Order Form... 167

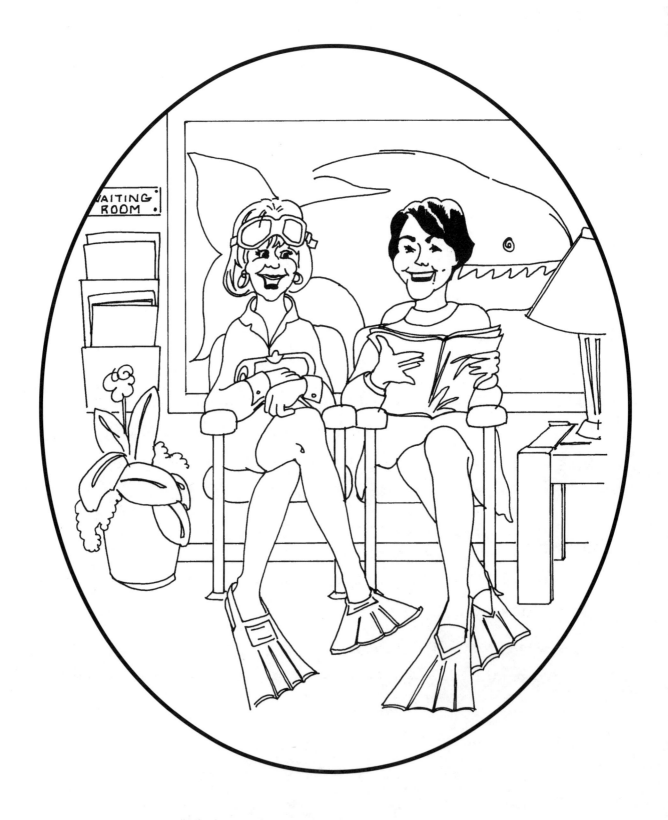

"I think you and I might have something in common."

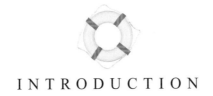

INTRODUCTION

Strategies of Survival

Cancer S.O.S.: **Strategies of Survival** is a guidebook, written for women who must battle cancer by women who have battled cancer. Cancer is about survival, and the road to survival is knowledge and hope. The purpose of this book is to provide you with both, in an informative, understandable and realistic format. This book is intended to be read after your diagnosis — right after! We have written the book in practical language so as not to overwhelm you. Your diagnosis has already done that, and we want to take some of the mystery and terror out of that diagnosis. Step by step, we will take you through the cancer survival process, giving you the information you need to take control of your disease, your treatment, and your life. We've included worksheets at the end of each chapter to assist you through each step of the cancer survival process, as well as resource guides and a glossary to explain all the medical terms that will be thrown your way without the benefit of an interpreter.

This is your workbook. Use a pencil, pen, marker or even a crayon to fill in the worksheets. They are to go with you to the doctor or hospital and should be filled out completely.

They <u>will</u> help you understand your cancer care and make your path easier to follow.

Before you begin reading, in the true spirit of introduction, we would like to tell you a little about ourselves. We are only slightly different versions of you.

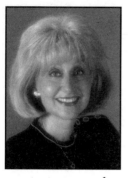

Rose

I have a cancer story that will frighten even the most well meaning listener. Unfortunately my story is similar to many other cancer patients. I had breast cancer in 1990, radical mastectomy, and seven surgeries later, full breast reconstruction. I had eight months of chemotherapy and survived to tell my story of how little the doctors knew about how to help a patient struggle through the mental and physical problems associated with my disease. I had five years of cancer free living and then was hit with Stage III ovarian cancer. I had spent months trying to convince my gynecologist and oncologist that something was wrong with me. Even though I had all the classic symptoms of ovarian cancer and a family history, they both felt I was under stress and imagining I had cancer. I finally took matters into my own hands and forced an oncologist to order a CAT scan. Lo and behold, ovarian cancer had spread all over my pelvic area. After debulking surgery, colon resections and chemotherapy I had one year of cancer-free living and fell out of remission. I am currently in remission after another round of chemotherapy.

My purpose in contributing to this book is to let you know there is a way to get through this and help you survive cancer.

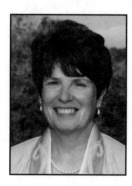

Shirley

My cancer experience began in December, 1991. My cancer arrived without symptoms, while I was feeling perfectly healthy and planning to live forever. A common blood test during a routine physical exam turned up an abnormality. The first fingers of fear crept into my life. Following more extensive blood tests and a bone marrow test, I was diagnosed with Acute Myelogenous Leukemia. Fear grabbed hold with an iron fist. I had a disease I could barely pronounce

that, even with treatment, had an extremely low survival rate. Without treatment, I would definitely die. I was hospitalized and began an induction treatment of 168 hours of uninterrupted chemotherapy, followed by four additional weeks of hospitalization, mostly in isolation, while my body worked through the effects of the chemo. Feeling fine became a distant memory. After three weeks of limited "freedom" at home, I returned to the hospital for two successive sessions of "consolidation chemotherapy". These were virtual repeats of the initial process, again separated by a three-week parole at home. Finally, for five months I had self-injected maintenance chemotherapy at home.

I am very fortunate. I achieved a strong first remission, and to date am doing very well. But it has been a long, tough road to get to the point where I am now. There is so much I did not know when I received my diagnosis; so much information that I needed but had no idea how to find. In retrospect, my ignorance of my own disease was appalling, and inexcusable. As a result of this ignorance, I learned many lessons the hard way. I don't want you to do the same. Neither does Rose. The result is this book.

The information compiled in the following chapters is designed to walk you through the cancer process. We may sound very firm in our convictions. We are. We have interviewed other cancer patients, doctors, nurses, and technicians and pulled from our own experiences. A lot of people have made this journey. They have generously shared their experiences and advice with us, that we may pass this knowledge on to you. Cancer is about survival. The road to survival is knowledge and hope. The purpose of this book is to provide you with both. We want you to survive. Please use our worksheets, make value decisions, and be a survivor.

We are not medically trained. Any suggestions we have made or references to medical treatment are based solely on our experiences or those related to us from other patients.

Please check with your doctor before you do anything other than your prescribed treatment.

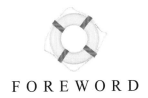

Walking in the Same Shoes

There are many serious diseases that affect the human condition, and challenge the beauty and comfort of our lives. None gives birth to images and fears so consistently as the disease we call cancer. The unfortunate reality is that a diagnosis of cancer has a profound affect not only on the patient, but also on her family and her entire circle of friends. Their lives all change as the day to day impact of diagnostic testing, treatment, recovery and follow-up evolve. A diagnosis of cancer does not come and go like a gallbladder attack, or pneumonia. A heart attack somehow seems more compatible with the continuation of one's life. Even when the diagnosis is made early, for many patients the cancer becomes a chronic disease, never quite going away, and always requiring some management. The patient is bound to a disease that will be in and out of her thoughts for years to come.

Patients today are much more informed about health care issues, and far more assertive on their own behalf. Long gone are the days when the typical patient would simply follow any directive from their doctor solely because he is the doctor. Patients have become more aware that the practice of medicine is often a sequence of judgments rather than the exact science we would like it to be. The search for more information often leading to alternative paths of therapy is commonly practiced by patients and their entire support system, who seek to partner in these judgments. Still at other times the patient is more comfortable leaving the therapeutic decisions solely to their doctor(s), and focusing their energy seeking a greater understanding of the changes in their life, and how they can cope more effectively. For the cancer patient, many of your new challenges are familiar to Rose Welsh and Shirley Grandahl for they have *"walked in your shoes"*. They have real credibility, for they have experienced what many of you have or will experience.

Cancer S.O.S.: Strategies of Survival is a highly practical resource that can make many somber days a bit lighter, and many hurdles a little bit lower. Your support system has just become stronger as you are accompanied through your diagnosis, the tests that often follow, and the treatment for your cancer. You will be given some "Do's and Don'ts", some advice on feeling good about yourself, and some specifics on nutrition and exercise. And then as if this were not enough for the best of support systems, a chapter on financial, insurance and legal concerns will come to your aid. The book also contains a useful glossary of medical terms, and a very practical resource guide (especially if you have access to a computer), that will add considerably to your confidence as a knowledgeable active participant in your care.

Rose and Shirley have found you, and you have found them. They have no doubt achieved great personal satisfaction from recording their experiences and then going far beyond by creating this *"guidebook for women with cancer"*. I'm quite confident that with them on your side, you'll stand taller and stronger as you face the challenges ahead. I wish you well.

Jerome L. Belinson M.D.
Chairman
Department of Gynecology and Obstetrics
The Cleveland Clinic Foundation

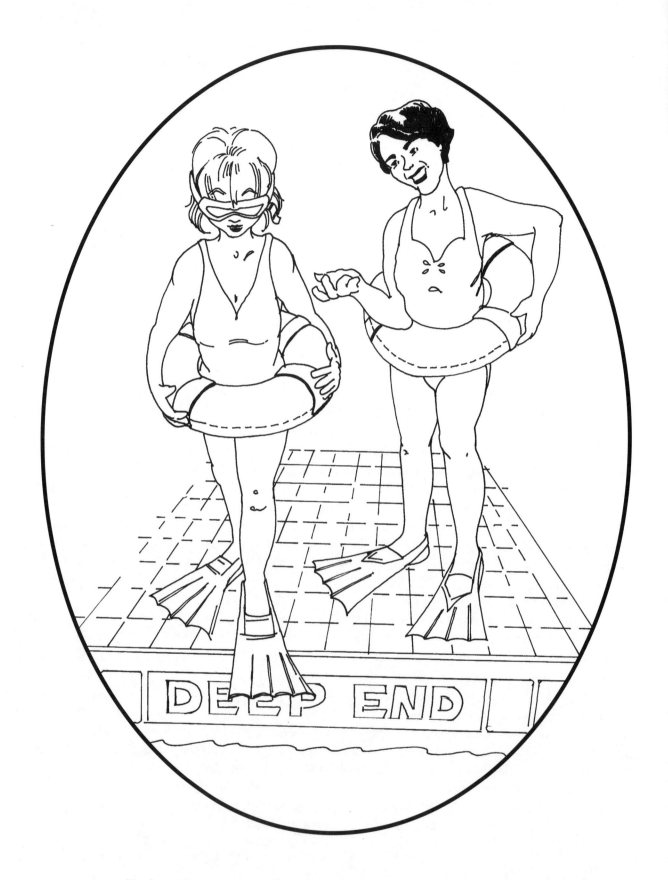

"Look at it this way... we really need more options than just 'Sink' or 'Swim'."

Strategy #1: Understanding Your Diagnosis

In the United States, women have a 1 in 3 lifetime risk of developing cancer. Cancer does not discriminate. Over a half-million new cancer cases in women are diagnosed each year. It is a dangerous opponent. When the doctor says, "I am afraid it's cancer", you are immediately at war. Your first battle is with your own devastated emotions, an overwhelming onslaught of feelings dominated by fear. You equate the diagnosis of cancer with death. It is quite likely that you did not hear much more of what the doctor said to you after the word cancer. You have already heard more than you can handle and your brain has temporarily gone into shutdown while it tries to relate the significance of this word "cancer" to your life. You are numb, angry and frightened. Thoughts like: "The doctor must be wrong; Maybe my tests were mixed up with those of someone else; Am I going to die?; Are they telling me everything?; This isn't happening; and I would really like to wake up from this nightmare right now!", are the usual reactions. Eventually, and probably too quickly for most of us, the facts sink in and we are left with the reality of cancer in our lives.

Now what do you do? First, rid yourself of that "death image". Cancer is not automatically a death sentence. The first thing you need to do is make an appointment to see the doctor again in a few days. Then go home and take some time to adjust to the news. Unless the doctor tells you that you have to act immediately, take a few days to absorb the shock. You may have to wait a few days for additional test results. These days will be the longest you have ever known. Use them to get yourself under control. If you want to win this war, you need time to learn about your adversary and prepare for battle.

The second thing you need to do is practice a concept that may be completely foreign to you: "put yourself first". This is an incredibly important philosophy that will prove essential to your well being in the immediate future.

I received this advice within days of my diagnosis. Judy Foster, a Clinical Nurse Specialist at Hartford Hospital and the Helen and Harry Gray Cancer Center in Hartford , Connecticut, took me aside and said those three very important words to me: "Put yourself first". That sounds pretty obvious and simplistic. But it isn't. Without realizing it, I was considering everyone else's feelings, and placing my own pretty far down on the ladder. How will my family deal with this? What is this going to do to the kids? How is my husband going to be able to manage our children, our home, his job, and now all the extra "burden" that I'm going to be? What about our insurance? Our income?

The list of my concerns was endless. I was concerned with the effect my illness was going to have on everyone else. Perhaps as a way to avoid focusing on what was about to happen to ME, I was totally focused on matters that I actually needed to hand over to others. Thankfully, from her experience and expertise in working with cancer patients, Judy sensed this. Her advice bears repeating: "Put yourself first!" — Shirley

---

Your mind is trying to cope with your diagnosis and is flooded with frightening thoughts. Express them. If you think that you must be courageous and fight this without releasing the flood of emotions that have filled you to the bursting point, think again. That isn't healthy. You need to take control over what will be happening to you in the coming months, and the best way to do that is to be honest with yourself, and good to yourself.

Don't put pressure on yourself to be brave and strong. You are brave and strong. To fight this formidable enemy takes enormous courage and energy. Don't waste your precious energy trying to "act brave". There are no cowards when it comes to cancer. Just fighting the disease takes more courage than most people will have to muster up in their whole lives. The secret to this battle is to break it down into little "skirmishes", one conflict at a time. Doing otherwise creates enormous additional stress.

Stress is detrimental to your immune system, which you need now more than ever. Stress can amplify the side effects of treatment and slow your recovery. Stress-relief techniques are essential to your treatment and recovery. Go for a walk. Listen to meditation tapes. Rely on whatever healthy stress-relief tactics work best for you!

I went jogging. I guess I thought I could run away from the news. Then I came home and cried - a lot. — Shirley

---

"Shirley's diagnosis came out of nowhere."

"We went from having our whole future ahead of us to total uncertainty, from health to horror. Shirley felt fine, and yet in a matter of days we had gone from "nothing wrong" to "terminal illness". I felt confused. I couldn't accept it.

I had difficulty adjusting to the fact that our life together had changed so swiftly. From biking and running to chemo and catheters! Our world now revolved around blood counts and fear. Technically, Shirley was the one with leukemia. But realistically, we had it. This battle was not hers alone, it was ours."

- Russ (Shirley's husband)

4

The third time I heard that cancer news I was really scared. I went through all of the emotion stages again. I started with fear, went to anger and right back to fear again. I was so scared. I cried at the thought of facing treatment again. I couldn't sleep. I was a wreck. I knew I had to deal with the cancer or die, so I got all the tears, screams and tantrums out of my system in a week or so and dug my heels in to make another stand. — Rose

Accepting your emotions and dealing with your stress will allow you to channel your energy toward positive action. Put your energy into becoming organized and well informed. Gathering information about your illness may seem like a monumental task that you are not capable of tackling right now, but you have to. It is essential to your survival. Knowledge is your road to a better quality of life. You must take an active part in your treatment and recovery.

Work on harnessing your fear. Fear is your enemy. It will cause you to make dangerous mistakes, uninformed decisions, and disrupt what little normalcy is left in your life. You have a very big responsibility; *you have to save your life.* Dr. Bernie S. Siegel has published several books that should be mandatory reading for all people with serious illnesses! Both "Love, Medicine, & Miracles" and "Peace, Love & Healing" are incredible sources of help, teaching you about self-healing. Dr. Siegel's tapes, "How to Live Between Office Visits" are fortified with encouragement and hope and will give you courage to keep on going.

Right after I was diagnosed, I had a terrible time keeping my wits about me. Each night rather than scream myself to sleep, I listened to Dr. Bernie Siegel on his "Healing Meditations" tape. I cried each night at the imagery and the wonderful peace his soothing words gave me. I actually felt God was with me on my mind journey. When the tape clicked off each night, I would drift off to sleep thinking how WELL I was going to be. The next morning I awoke refreshed and ready for the mountain of problems that would be thrown at me that day. Every time I felt the burden was too great, I tuned in on my headphones and tuned out the problems. I recommend the tape. In fact, I think it is an integral part of your survival kit. There is more information in this book on how to find Dr. Siegel's tapes. They're one of the best investments in peace of mind that you can make. — Rose

"In September of 1995 the fears of the previous year became reality in a waiting room of the Miami Heart Institute."

"The request to follow the doctor into the Patients' Consultation room only confirmed what Rose and I had known for the previous nine months and had been unable to convince two oncologists and a gynecologist. The pain in her lower abdomen, the bloating and constipation were not "stress-related or imagined", but were indeed caused by a malignancy. It was ovarian cancer!"

- Gary (Rose's Husband)

Should you tell the whole family? It is your decision. Generally, you won't be able to hide it from those you live with, or see and talk to frequently. Cancer is a lonely illness, and we highly recommend that you do not try to bear it alone.

You will need to decide how to tell your family. This is very definitely a personal issue. Remember that, just like you, your family will need time to work out their feelings about your diagnosis. Do not spend time trying to console them. You must be concerned about your own emotional and physical health. When you feel like you are in control yourself, then you can help your family. In the meantime they need to settle this news in their own minds.

Older family members may be physically fragile, but they can be wonderfully strong when times get tough. They have experienced life's joys and sorrows and know how to deal with difficult situations. So don't feel you must protect them. Children actually cope with sickness better when they have been given an explanation of your illness. Young children may not need a clinical explanation, but if they are told that Mom or Grandma is sick and are given a brief description of the changes they may expect , it will quiet some of their fears.

My two-year-old granddaughter, Madeline, liked me to spin my wig around. I was her only Gramma that could take her hair off. She loved that and always wanted me to show everyone how I did it. — Rose

---

Life might change for you and your family, but it may mean only minor adjustments. Don't imagine the worst.

Everyone may have to assume different roles for awhile, but that should be good for them! Feeling useful helps people cope. This is your opportunity to get some help in the kitchen and form some really nice new family habits! Not that we suggest that you take advantage of the situation, but imagine yourself on the couch with the TV remote in your hand while your family makes, and yes, cleans up the dinner mess. Picture them vacuuming. Picture them cleaning the bathroom. This is really healthful imagery.

This might be a good time to call a friend or family member and talk to them. The best person to talk to is someone who has had cancer. They can help you through these early days when all seems so over-whelming. No matter whom you choose let someone else know how you feel. Most friends and family will rally around you. It is an opportunity for them to show you how much they love you.

There are so many issues ahead to deal with. Your family and friends can take the burden of some of these problems from you. Begin to create a circle of love and support around yourself. This circle will sustain you in the days to come.

When I came home from the hospital, I had lost quite a bit of weight. I thought I looked pretty good; a tough way to diet, but a diet none-the-less. My prognosis was questionable; however, my attitude was great. When friends would stop by to see how I was doing, some would cry, some would turn away because I had changed in physical appearance. It frightened them. However the visits were good for all of us. I think my good attitude actually made them feel better about me and about them-selves too. Those first brave souls who stopped by are the ones that stayed by me throughout my recovery. — Rose

---

In some cases, friends and family members seem to disappear when they hear the news. It is not because they don't care, but more likely that they are afraid for you and don't know what to say. Or it may be that your illness has made them more aware of their own mortality and they have difficulty facing you because they are frightened for themselves. So often, they just need time to adjust to your news and will soon be back to rejoin your circle of support.

Expect some changes at work. Co-workers often feel awkward talking to you when you are sick. It is entirely possible that you will look and feel almost the same as you do now. Your treatment may only keep you out of work for a few days or weeks. You may be so much like your pre-cancer self that everyone at work will actually forget you are ill. However, some cancer treatment is aggressive and can make you feel sick, look unwell, and keep you from your job for an extended period of time. Your boss may be worried that you won't come back to work, or may become concerned about how long he will have to hold your job until you are well enough to come back. There are

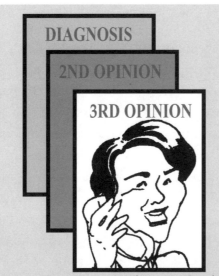

Let your emotions work with your mind. You would shop around for carpeting and all you are going to do is walk on it, so why accept the first doctor who comes up with a treatment plan? Treatments vary from doctor to doctor, hospital to hospital, and state to state. Make the time to place a few long distance calls.

ways to deal with this issue. We discuss employment issues in Chapter Seven.

With my second bout with cancer, I was out of work for six weeks. My boss, Harry, was great. He asked someone from the office to call me each day to say hello. It was especially great for me, but I think it was also good for everyone at the office. I felt I was still part of the crew, and they could hear how much like my old self I was! — Rose

Everyone copes with stressful situations a little differently. They may be waiting for you to show them how to act around you. This is an uncomfortable time for all concerned. Don't be too critical. Most people eventually "come around". You will be very busy and may not even notice their absence. Or it may be that friends don't come and you have to go it alone, or are deserted by some of your loved ones. It is sad to think of how unhappy they will be some day when they realize how they treated you. But that is their burden, not yours.

Whether you have a strong support system or not, there are other places to turn for a warm, friendly hug. If you are a member of a church or temple, the members of your faith can offer you enormous support. Cancer support groups are abundant and extremely helpful. Nearly all cancer treatment centers sponsor support groups. Also, the American Cancer Society offers support groups for patients and families. Call 1-800-ACS-2345 for the ACS division nearest you, or find the location and phone number in the appendix at the end of this book. The American Cancer Society staff can direct you to a support group in your area. Support groups are run by facilitators, professionals in the medical field trained to work with cancer patients and their families. The atmosphere is friendly, relaxed and comforting. It is enormously helpful to talk with other people who are sharing your experience.

While I was in the hospital undergoing treatment, my husband began attending a support group for patients and their families sponsored by the Leukemia Society of America. He found it helpful and informative. It gave him an opportunity to share his feelings, his fears, his problems, and to learn more about my disease. The hospital I was in held "in-house" support meetings for the patients on the oncology floor. Talking with others who are walking in your "hospital slippers" is enormously beneficial to your feelings of hope and well being. — Shirley

---

A quick tip: This is no time to be listening to horror stories about how "my aunt's cousin had a terrible time with her cancer", followed by a detailed description of her colostomy problems. Ask anyone, and we do mean anyone, who has negative information, a negative attitude, or negative comments to get out of your presence and don't come back until they have something positive to say. Your mental attitude right now is critical to your future. Much of the anxiety you are feeling is fear of the unknown. You need to defray some of the stress you are experiencing.

Spirituality may be your key to peace of mind. This may be the time to have a good one-on-one talk with God. If you have not been a faithful follower, you may feel guilty asking God to make you well. Remember He hears your prayers and like the Prodigal Son, will take you back. Search your soul and come to your own decision on your relationship with God. Your religious beliefs and prayers may offer great consolation to you. This is a personal choice.

Try meditation. It works. There are many books, tapes and classes available on meditation. It is easy to learn and well worth the effort. You need to regain control of your mind and body. Regaining your peace of mind may seem difficult. You need full control of your mind if you want to have control over your body.

Both meditation and visualization are *easy-to-learn* techniques that work wonderfully. You may very well be a disbeliever, as both of us were. But you are in for a big and pleasant surprise.

Meditation may sound like something done only in the presence of the Dali Lama, but it really is a comforting mind-calming exercise that will help put the situation in perspective. Visualization is almost fun. It is a way to put your thoughts into positive action. You could be sitting in a beach chair looking at the ocean and both meditating and visualizing.

Sound great? It can be.
If you are anxious to get started
Chapter Six will give you a beginner's
course. You can take it from there.

Many times during the course of my illness I would close my eyes and picture myself sitting under a spreading banyan tree in a lush forest and see Jesus standing over me with his hand on my shoulder. I knew He was there with me and I felt great peace. When I opened my eyes I was ready for any challenge. I was not alone. — Rose

An Important Reminder:

A few things to remember in these early, frightening days:

- Cancer is not synonymous with death.

- A diagnosis is a forecast, a prediction, an OPINION.

- Many severe cancers are curable.

- You can and must control your situation.

- You are not alone. Support is out there for the asking.

- You have choices. You need not follow blindly.

- Pay no attention to statistics. You are not a number.

Survival statistics are based on averages. Five Year Survival Rates are averages collected by researchers and hospitals.

Here is the Real Deal. Trials may run over a five year span, say 1985 - 1990. By the time they are published, say in 1995, the lag time makes the numbers somewhat invalid.

Even the most recently released data on survival prognosis is dated enough so as not to reflect the latest advances in treatment. Also, some studies do not take into account the varying ages and health of patients at the time of diagnosis and treatment.

This is why we say:

"Don't pay attention to statistics."

"I don't think of all the misery, but of all the beauty that still remains."
- Anne Frank

"Keep your face to the sunshine and you cannot see the shadows."
- Helen Keller

"In God I will praise his word, in God I have put my trust; I will not fear what flesh can do unto me."
- Psalm 56:4

What Am I Dealing With?

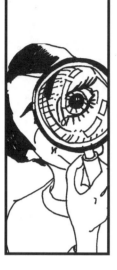

What is cancer? Cancer is a large group of diseases, over 100 different conditions marked by the uncontrolled growth and spread (metastasis) of abnormal cells. If cancer is not controlled, it almost always ends in death. Obviously, this is your cue — *get it under control*.

How is it treated? Cancer can be treated in many different ways. Doctors may recommend surgery, chemotherapy, radiation, or biological therapy. Unconventional treatments can range from laetrile to castor oil wraps. We do not endorse any particular treatment. You must choose what you feel is best for you after you have researched your condition. The National Cancer Institute recommends conventional treatments. Call the Cancer Info Line at 1-800-4-CAN-CER. For information on other available treatments go to the library, to health professionals, or search the Internet's World Wide Web. Alternative therapies are available to you. Look in health food store magazines, investigate metabolic physicians. Be careful not to put your faith in an unproved treatment just because it sounds more palatable than conventional treatment. To make the right decision you must *Be Informed*.

"Question Authority."
- Bernie S. Siegel, M.D.

What do I do next? By now a physician has recommended that you see an oncologist. This is a good idea. HOWEVER, there are many types of oncologists out there. If your diagnosis is breast cancer, find an oncologist who specializes in breast cancer. A diagnosis of ovarian cancer demands that a doctor who treats mainly ovarian cancer patients treats you. Oncologists generally see many types of patients; some with breast, uterine or ovarian cancers, some with melanoma, cancer of the brain, liver, or lung, and leukemia. They cannot possibly be current on the latest treatments for all cancers.

Compare this to your car; would you take your Rolls Royce to a Yugo mechanic for repair? Of course not. This is your body, you're the Rolls, and it is your life that is on the line. Find a doctor that is treating your type of cancer in great numbers. He will have the experience you need.

(Authors' note: When referring to physicians by pronoun, we realized that we needed to be gender-consistent, and while the pronoun 'it' seemed the least sexist, we decided after much deliberation to use the masculine pronoun. We wish to make it clear, however, that although we are using the masculine, we are really referring to physicians of both genders!)

Doctors vary in training, experience and services. These differences become very important when you are looking for the best possible treatment for your condition. Doctors who are board-certified have completed training in their specialty as outlined by the American Board of Medical Specialties, practiced for a specified time period, and passed difficult examinations in their specialty areas. Some specialties do not have specific certification. A breast surgeon may be certified in general surgery. Find an oncologist who is board certified and is a specialist in your cancer treatment. This is the person you want heading up your team.

It takes a team. Don't be lulled into the Comfort Zone by thinking that one doctor is the answer to your problem. Actually, if you are to get well, wouldn't you rather have many minds focused on your cure, rather than just one? A team of health professionals may include an oncologist, radiologist, cancer surgeon, pathologist, and a nutritionist. They can discuss and agree on a treatment plan and customize a program for your particular cancer problem.

Choosing the right doctor and hospital may make a huge difference in the quality of your life during recovery. Do not forget to include yourself on the team! In fact, think of yourself as the quarterback or the coach. You will be calling the plays. If you don't, you will find yourself out of the game before the starting whistle blows.

Your Team of Cancer Specialists:

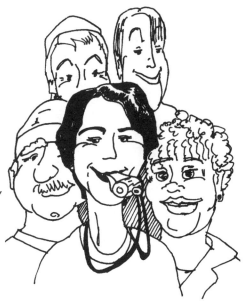

Cancer Surgeon: A surgeon with training and experience in removing tumors and repairing organs damaged by cancer. Your survival is based on his ability.

Nurse Practitioner: A nurse who has completed the RN degree plus additional highly specialized training. She may work with or without the supervision of a physician, and take on additional duties in diagnosis and treatment of patients. In many states, she may write prescriptions. (See also Oncology Nurse Specialist)

Oncologist: A physician specializing in the treatment of cancer. Some of the specialists within this field include:
- **Gynecologic - Oncologist:** specializes in treating diseases of the female reproductive organs
- **Hematology - Oncologist:** treats leukemia, lymphoma, multiple myeloma, and Hodgkin's Disease
- **Medical Oncologist:** treats cancers by means of drugs and chemotherapy
- **Neurosurgeon:** specializes in surgery on the brain and other parts of the nervous system
- **Radiation Oncologist:** treats cancer with external and internal radiation
- **Diagnostic Oncologist:** interprets x-rays and scans to pinpoint cancers

Doctor of Internal Medicine: Internist who specializes in care of cancer patients.

Nutritionist: An expert in nutrition, especially the series of processes by which an organism (in this case, you!) takes in and assimilates food for promoting growth and replacing worn or injured tissues.

Oncology Nurse Specialist: A nurse who has taken specialized training in the field of cancer, after completing the registered nurse (RN) degree. Many oncology nurses are also certified nurse practitioners.

Pathologist: Physician who specializes in the identification of abnormalities and disease by examining tissue under a microscope.

Therapist: Medical personnel specially trained in care and treatment of disease. Ex.: an Enterostomal Therapy Nurse, also known as an ET nurse, is trained to take care of and teach ostomy patients.

Remember: Build a strong, positive relationship with your caregivers. Ask questions and be informed.

Interview your doctors.

You can do this on the phone if you like, but we suggest you meet them in person if possible. Request a copy of your test results and take them with you when speaking with the physician. *If he is not thoroughly committed to helping you, if his attitude is complacent, if you are at all uncomfortable with the doctor, go somewhere else!* Your treatment could be worth upwards of $250,000 to the doctor. You should be really convinced that this is the health professional to help you. You are entrusting your life to this physician's care, so be absolutely sure you have confidence in the doctor's ability and commitment to getting you well again.

When evaluating and selecting your physician remember that a warm and comforting bedside manner is important, but MAY NOT equate to a competent professional. To be completely sure, you can check on your doctor by calling your state's Health Services Department. This state department will give you information about the physician's schooling, board certification, license status, and any claims, charges or allegations that may have been made against him. (This info may not be easy to get, but be persistent.)

Your county medical society will also give you information about a doctor's education, license, board-certification, age, and hospital affiliation. This kind of background check may seem a little paranoid, but it is something to consider. However, please remember that charges made against a physician may not be valid. Frivolous lawsuits are not exactly uncommon!

Cancer care is serious business and you want and deserve only the very best!

Recently, the nightly news brought this message home rather soberly. It reported on a physician service, contracted by a legitimate Texas hospital, which performed over 800 surgeries in a six-month period with personnel not licensed as physicians. The so-called doctors were not accredited. Some had degrees from foreign schools, but the majority were not licensed. The state had to research all surgeries that were performed, solely or assisted, by the group to determine negligence and/or wrongful death! So don't be afraid to question everyone who comes near you, and if you are not comfortable with their answers or behavior, investigate.

Get three opinions.

Doctors can view your illness in many ways, including incorrectly. Ask for your records and tests; they are just that — yours. Educate yourself on your illness and become an expert in your care. When you speak to the doctors, know something about your particular condition. This tactic is a great filter. If you have knowledge, he will have to respond in the same manner. If he is lacking in new information, that should tell you to get out and find someone who knows at least as much as you do! You can get information from the American Cancer Society, the library, bookstores, hospital libraries, universities, research centers, the National Cancer Institute at 1/800-4-CANCER, the Internet, and local hospitals. Send your records to the best facilities available and ask the head of the department for a consultation.

Most insurance companies pay for a second opinion. The third may be on you. Spend the money. Remember you do not have to limit yourself to the city in which you live.

Let your emotions work with your mind. You would shop around for carpeting and all you are going to do is walk on it, so why accept the first doctor who comes up with a treatment plan? Treatments vary from doctor to doctor, hospital to hospital, and state to state. Make a few long-distance calls. It doesn't take long to gather this information. In less than a week you can have life-saving news in your hands.

At the end of this chapter you will find a worksheet we have developed for you to take with you when selecting an oncologist. Make copies and use it each time you talk to a prospective oncologist. Please take the time to be selective. After you have filled it out three or more times, sit down and evaluate the physicians using their answers and the feelings you got when you interviewed them. Staff and commitment cannot be evaluated solely on paper.

We know this is a lot of work, but keep at it. It's Important!

13

In, Florida, the oncologist who received my files from my gynecologist, read my test results and told me that I had Stage III ovarian cancer. My survival chances were minimal. He did say he had one patient that lived five years. I felt lost and called my brother in Ohio who suggested I contact the Cleveland Clinic. The Clinic is a world-renown facility most notably acclaimed for heart transplantation. I was frightened, but thought I should give it a try. I met with the chairperson of the Surgical Oncology Department. He evaluated my records, suggested immediate surgery, and when all was done, said he had removed over 90% of the cancer and I had a great chance for recovery. See what a second opinion can do for you? This doctor and his staff treated breast and ovarian cancers regularly and saw many successful patients. — Rose

OK, I've interviewed the doctors. Now what?

This is where it gets more complicated. You have received opinions from all the doctors you have spoken with. Now you have to decide which opinion you want to go with. (Remember: OPINIONS are judgment calls). A human being gives an opinion based on his experience. However, each cancer and each patient are different. There is no way to definitively predict the outcome. You will probably have as much to do with the outcome as the doctor will. So you need to choose the doctor whose credentials, attitude, personal demeanor, and judgment of your case you are most comfortable with. You must have a good relationship with your doctor. Once you have found an oncologist you have confidence in, work to keep your relationship strong, open and active.

As we said, treatments do vary. Make sure you are receiving the best. Medical personnel, doctors, nurses, and technicians can do terrible mental damage to you with a negative comment. Please get away from anyone who is not positively on your team. An oncologist who is committed to keeping you alive offers hope for your future. Hope will give you the strength to fight back. Do not let anyone, including your doctor, take that away from you.

How can you choose the right medical facility? There are many indicators that can be evaluated when making this decision. According to a report, "The Quality of Medical Care: Information for Consumers", published by the U.S. Congress, Office of Technology Assessment, you need to combine the information from more than one indicator. Patients about to have surgery for cancer can be more confident if a hospital performs a high number of these surgical procedures, has a low surgical mortality rate, and if the surgeon has extensive training and experience in the procedure. **Clearly, if the hospital has a high mortality rate and low volume of the procedure... RUN!**

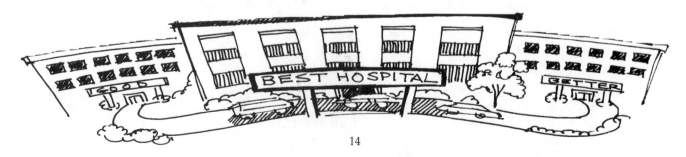

According to the 1989 December issue of "New England Journal of Medicine", private, not-for-profit teaching hospitals have a lower mortality rate than other types of hospitals.

"Ideally, the individuals engaged in patient care, research and teaching are organized around a given disease or class of patients, facilitating the sharing of knowledge, research and clinical findings. This results in an important interchange of ideas between laboratory, researchers and clinical practitioners, so that what happens in the laboratory influences what happens in clinical practice, and vice versa.

Ultimately, this approach results in the most rapid transfer of basic scientific knowledge from the laboratory to care delivery at the patient's bedside."

The Cleveland Clinic in Cleveland, Ohio recommends that when choosing a cancer treatment center you evaluate the facility's:

✗ *credentials*

✗ *experience*

✗ *range of services*

✗ *participation in research and education*

✗ *patient satisfaction*

✗ *outcome*

Other factors may need to be considered also. How important is it to you to be treated close to home? Will travel be a problem? The religious affiliation of a treatment center may also be of importance to you. The important thing is that the doctors and the center are the best you can find. Read the questions and information on our Hospital Worksheet at the end of this chapter and use the worksheet. It will help you choose the facility that is best for you. (We mention the Cleveland Clinic, but there are many excellent cancer treatment centers across the United States, Canada and around the world. We have listed NCI Cancer Centers in the U.S. in the Appendix section.)

Cancer is big business, and it's treatment expensive. Your medical insurance should pay for part of your treatment costs. Be sure to check with your insurance carrier about policy terms, limitations, stipulations and other requirements. Also, the cancer center that you choose will be able to help you with insurance matters and direct you to organizations that may be able to assist you with other financial concerns related to your treatment. Chapter Seven will be helpful in deciphering the insurance hieroglyphics.

What if I choose a treatment center out of my area?

If you choose or require treatment at a cancer center out of your area, there are volunteer organizations that can arrange for transportation to these medical facilities. **Angel Flight's** volunteer pilots can fly you from your home to treatment centers, allowing you easy and economical access to the ultimate care. Angel Flight is located in many U.S. states and can be found by contacting **NPATH: the National Patient Air Transport Hotline** at 1-800-296-2917. **Air Life Line of Sacramento, California**, offers transportation, and if they cannot help you, they will refer you to someone who can. You can contact them at 1-800-446-1231. **Air Care Alliance** is a nationwide association of humanitarian flying organizations, including **Angel Flight, Mercy Medical Airlift, Wings of Freedom, Flights for Life, Lifeline Pilots, Mercy Med Flights**, and numerous others dedicated to community service which help needy patients fly to facilities to receive medical attention. They have flown over 24,000 patients to and from treatment centers since 1990. Call them at 1-800-296-1217. **Corporate Angels Network (CAN)** matches dates and destinations nationwide to find transportation for patients. Patients/families need to contact CAN three weeks before the scheduled appointment. CAN will try to match arrivals and departures from within 100 miles of your home and your destination. There is no guarantee of transportation both ways, so to be sure, they recommend that you buy tickets on commercial airlines. However, CAN has agreements with several airlines to refund or reissue unused tickets without penalty for patients. CAN tells patients to be prepared for them to call you within days of the scheduled flight with corporate travel possibilities. Call CAN at 1-914-328-1313. (The telephone numbers, plus applicable web site addresses for these organizations are listed in the appendix of the book.)

> **Angel Flight**
> **NPATH: the National Patient Air Transport Hotline**
> **1-800-296-2917.**
>
> **Air Life Line of Sacramento, California**
> **1-800-446-1231**
>
> **Air Care Alliance**
> **1-800-296-1217.**
>
> **Corporate Angels Network (CAN)**
> **1-914-328-1313**

Try not to worry about the money aspects. There are some helpful ideas in Chapter Seven that will work for you. Right now, the only thing that matters is getting and staying well. Use the Hospital Work Sheet at the end of this chapter to help you choose a health care facility. This is a critical decision. Be very serious in your endeavors.

USE THE WORKSHEETS THAT FOLLOW. MAKE THREE COPIES (AT LEAST) AND MAKE NO DECISIONS UNTIL YOU HAVE COMPLETED THEM. REVIEW EACH QUESTION AND COMPARE THE ANSWERS. MAKE AN INFORMED DECISION.

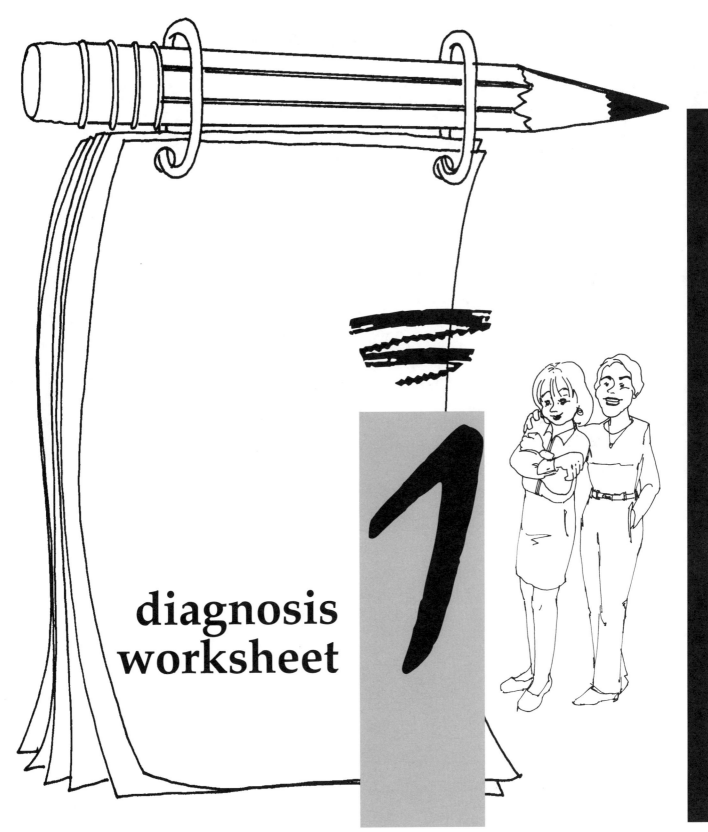

diagnosis
worksheet

1

diagnosis worksheet

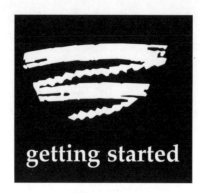

getting started

Τhis is a tough sheet to fill out. You must take an objective look at your illness. You must remain detached, as if it were someone else you were discussing. I'm sure you must think this is completely impossible, but you can do it. It is your chance to make a qualified decision about your future health. If you feel you are not capable of handling this, ask a friend or family member to help. This is a difficult and seemingly overwhelming task.

The diagnosis should be discussed with optimism. If it is not, stop the discussion and find another candidate. Truth can be delivered with hope.

You must be determined in asking the following questions. Your chances for long-term survival depend on you making the right decisions. Understand and be prepared to participate in your treatment. To do this you must know what you are up against.

Do not be afraid to ask questions. We know — you hate to upset the doctor. You are afraid he will be mad if you question his decisions. Well, he is making decisions that effect your future. If you feel bad you can go back and apologize after he makes you well.

Use this form to help develop your battle plan. Make copies and use it for each of your three opinions.

My diagnosis is:

~~~ What did the tests/biopsy show?

~~~ What exactly does that mean?   What is your opinion of my
      condition? *(If he feels there is little hope, STOP HERE,
      and get out of there. If you do not feel his commitment
      is to get you well, LEAVE NOW and find someone else).*

~~~ What parts of my body are affected?

~~~ Which parts can be affected?

~~~ What are my options as you see them?

~~~ How do you plan to make me well again?

~ Explain all of the plans you have for my recovery?

~ What is the treatment? Please be specific.

~ How long will it take?

~ What should I expect from the treatment?

~ How will it change my daily routine?

~ How often and for how long are the treatments?

~ What tests and procedures will be used to monitor my progress?

—⟋⟍— What research is being done? Where?

—⟋⟍— Where else can I get an opinion? *(If he tells you his opinion is the only one you need, he is wrong. If he can't suggest anyone, call the Cancer Information Service at 1/800 - 4 CANCER.)*

—⟋⟍— Do I need to see more than one doctor? *(Different types of specialists?)*

—⟋⟍— What other type of doctor should I see?

—⟋⟍— Would you consider working with a team of doctors?

—⟋⟍— When do you plan to start?

oncologist worksheet

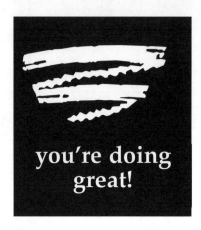

you're doing great!

〜〜 Are you Board Certified?

〜〜 How do you keep up with the latest procedures?

〜〜 Are you affiliated with a cancer RESEARCH center? Which one?

〜〜 Are you doing any research or trials on my type of cancer?

〜〜 Who is?

〜〜 Have you ever recommended a patient for a clinical trial?

〜〜 Does your office offer nutritional support?

~~~ How do you feel about complimentary medical treatment?
   (Acupuncture, massage, nutrition therapy)

~~~ Will you be consulting with other cancer professionals on my case?
   (If he doesn't answer, "Yes"- end the conversation. You don't need a "hot-dog" loner.)

~~~ How many patients with my type of cancer have you treated?

~~~ May I talk to a couple of them? If yes, what are their phone numbers?

~~~ What do you feel is my prognosis? *(This is a tough question because the answer may be a bitter pill to swallow. This is, however, the most important question you will ask this prospective physician. His response will allow you to look into the future and see if he plans to help you live or allows you to die. What you are looking for is some thing to the effect of: "My job is to make you well again. We'll work together towards that goal.")*

— How do I reach you in an emergency?

— What is your call policy?

— Who takes your calls when you are not in, or off for the weekend?

— What are his qualifications?

— Can I meet him? *(There is nothing worse than a panicky trip to the emergency room and then not being able to reach your trusted doctor!)*

— How much do you charge for treatment and follow-up?

— Can you bill me for only what my insurance pays?

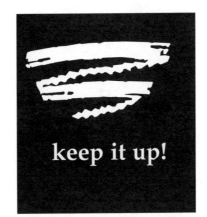

keep it up!

Note: Many hospitals report patient outcomes. Ask the hospital to provide its patient outcome information concerning cancer care. Be sure the information is adjusted to account for the severity of the illnesses of the patient population. If a hospital will not give you this information, get out and find a hospital that will.

⟋⟋⟋ Is this a teaching hospital?

⟋⟋⟋ Has the Joint Commission on Accreditation of Healthcare Organizations (JCAHO) accredited this hospital? If not, why not? (*Ask for the hospital's report card. Hospitals are rated by number (ex. 90%). You can call JCAHO to inquire about a hospital at 708/916-5800.*)

⟋⟋⟋ Does the Oncology department have a multi-disciplinary team approach?
Explain:

⟋⟋⟋ Would you consider your capabilities and equipment state of the art? Please give me examples that pertain to my situation.

⟋⟋⟋ Can I get a tour of the hospital and see its latest diagnostic equipment, treatment facilities, emergency room, and patient rooms?

—⁓⁓— Has the hospital been regularly recognized for medical excellence?

—⁓⁓— Does this hospital offer me access to experimental treatments through clinical trials?

—⁓⁓— What are your cancer survivor rates?

—⁓⁓— Explain the range of services offered?

—⁓⁓— Are your oncologist and team members certified in their specialties?

—⁓⁓— Does the hospital participate in clinical trials or cancer research? What kind of trials?

—⁓⁓— Would I have access to those trials if I need experimental treatments?

—⁓⁓— Do you keep patient satisfaction reports on patients? On employees? May I see them? *(Employee reports are important. If the staff is not happy, they quit. High turnover can affect quality of care and experience levels).*

~ How many patients with my type of cancer have you treated in the last couple of years?

~ Is there a program for patients and families to help us all get through this situation?

~ Tell me about your state-of-the-art diagnostic capabilities.

~ Will you begin discharge planning upon admission? *(This is very important for continuity of overall care. You don't want to have any gaps in your recovery and care process.)*

~ Will the tests and treatments be performed during the day? *(Many hospitals schedule outpatient tests during daytime hours and test hospital patients at night.)*

~ What are the policies regarding visiting hours? Can my family/friends come to see me whenever I/they want to?

~ Does the hospital use a lot of agency nurses? If so, do the nurses have long-term, progressive experience in cancer care? Explain how.

~ What is your policy on cancer care training for the staff?

~m~ Does the hospital offer home care services, including medical equipment?

~m~ Does the hospital conduct weekly tumor-board meetings to keep physicians updated on the latest cancer treatments?

~m~ Is the hospital affiliated with any other cancer care facilities? (*Many hospitals are part of large holding companies that have sister facilities throughout the U.S., like Loma Linda, Duke, or Sloan Kettering. You may want to avail yourself of their services.*)

~m~ Does the hospital have a pain management program? (*This is a designated department that specializes in keeping you as comfortable and pain-free as possible.*)

~m~ Is there a hospitality facility affiliated with the hospital for my friends and family members to stay at?

Strategy #2: Getting All The Facts

The doctors will want to run a barrage of tests on you and your many body parts. Learn what each test is and what it is designed to monitor or register. Learn which tests are used to diagnose your specific illness and be sure that the doctor is running them.

Do not expect the doctor to know or remember everything about you. In the last chapter you made a concentrated effort to determine the best team of health care providers. This is not the time to fall back and expect the team to carry you. You must understand what is happening to your body and how best to treat your illness. Your cancer is different from the next patient's cancer. Do not take a test without a full explanation of what it is for, how it is done, and how the results will apply to your treatment. Keep records of your tests to compare results and monitor your progress.

To help you track your progress, put together a notebook of your tests and results. If you feel you want another test performed, discuss it with your doctor. Be sure the test is necessary and will accomplish a goal, either yours or your doctor's. Keep the lines of communication open and know what is being done, or not done, to get you well. Tests are not fun, but they are needed to get a clear picture of what is happening in your body.

The worksheets at the back of this chapter are to be copied and taken with you when you visit your doctor or hospital. Make sure you understand every facet of the procedures. You are paying for every test, technician, and laboratory evaluation, etc. It is your life and your money.

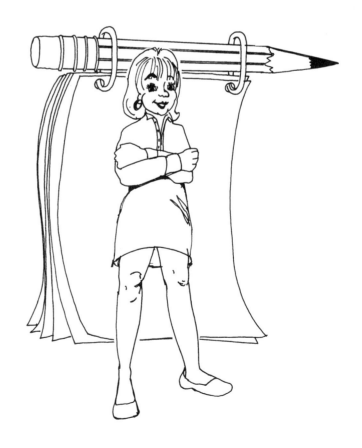

Take charge.

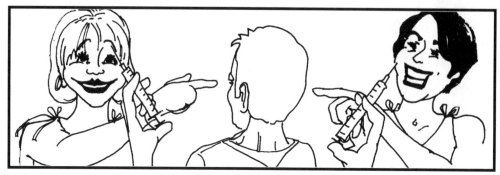

Following is a list of some of the more common tests. They are rated on something we call:

Rose and Shirley's Discomfort Scale
1 = painless, 10 = OUCH!

(Scores are based on personal experience, research, and input from other patients. Individual pain and discomfort may vary depending on the patient and the medical personnel administering the test. The scores are intended to give you a benchmark.)

Angiogram

1 An x-ray of blood vessels. Dye is injected and an x-ray is taken of the specific area. Painless, we rate this a 1 on the discomfort scale.

Aspiration Curettage

1.5 Tissue samples are removed through a tube connected to a surgical vacuum, not unlike your Hoover. This is usually done in the doctor's office. This one rates about a 1.5.

Barium Enema

2 Barium sulfate is dripped slowly into the rectum and colon to look for growths or other problems. This test is a little embarrassing, slightly uncomfortable, but really, only a 2.

Biopsy

1-4 A procedure in which tissue is taken and examined under a microscope by a pathologist.
Ex.: Needle Aspiration - A long, very thin needle is inserted into the tumor to remove a small tissue sample. This test is not routinely done with any anesthesia, which is unfortunate because while it is sometimes painless, in many instances it is unexpectedly painful. To be safe, we have to rate this one on a sliding scale of 1 - 4. You might want to discuss with your doctor the possibility of a little local anesthesia.

Blood Work

1-2 Your blood count is needed to sample and measure the number of white and red blood cells and platelets. It is a great diagnostic tool. You need to become familiar with the various types of blood tests, as they are used throughout your treatment to monitor your progress.

Before and after chemotherapy treatment, you will undergo various blood tests.

Blood is drawn from a vein, a port, or a central venous catheter (Hickman or Broviac). A port is a tube connected to a quarter-sized disc that is surgically placed just below the skin in the chest or abdomen. The tube is inserted into a large vein directly into the bloodstream. Blood products, fluids, and drugs can be infused and blood withdrawn through a needle inserted into the disc. You can refer to this as your own personal doorbell. A Hickman or Broviac catheter is special intravenous tubing that is surgically inserted into a large vein near the heart. The end of the catheter is tunneled under the skin and pulled out of an opening in the chest. You may feel like a cow attached to a milking machine; but the catheter, unlike a full set of udders, can be tucked nicely into your bra when not in use. As with the port, medication, fluids and blood products can be given through the catheter, and blood can be withdrawn. The ports and catheters are implanted while you have general anesthesia, in the operating room. You may experience some tenderness after the implant, but ultimately the catheter is painless. Neither one of these appliances are very attractive, but we, being clever women, learned to disguise these silly-looking yet helpful appliances with normal clothing.

Catheters require some maintenance. Every two to three days my Hickman catheter had to be flushed out with heparin to prevent clotting, and the site of the implant had to be thoroughly cleaned, disinfected and re-bandaged. My husband and I were trained by the hospital staff on how to do this. My husband did not particularly like doing this, but he did a terrific job. I never got any type of infection at the site of my catheter. Catheter infections are not uncommon. With that in mind, I wish to point out that although my doctors told me it was all right to take a shower while I had the Hickman in me, I got different advice from several nurses. A friend did a little research for me on the subject, and after considering all the information, I decided not to risk taking showers. There is no way to keep the dirty, soapy water from getting into the wound, and considering that the catheter goes directly into a large vein near the heart, I felt that it was just too easy for germs to gain access to my body through this portal to my circulatory system. With a battered immune system, this did not seem like such a good idea, and I felt the risk was too great. I chose to take sponge baths. With no body hair to worry about, it was quick, easy and safe. And, most importantly, I was clean! — Shirley

---

The port and the central venous catheter provide for less painful infusion of necessary fluids and withdrawal of blood for frequent testing. However, even if your blood test requires insertion of a needle, the pain factor is low. If you are squeamish, MAKE the nurse or blood technician use a small needle. Pain all gone!

1-2.5 CBC (Complete Blood Count)

Blood tests are painless if you have a port or catheter; and only moderately uncomfortable if you have to be poked. Depending on your pain threshold, and supply of nice juicy veins, these tests can range anywhere from a 1 to a 2.5. Usually, it's a one. The most common test ordered is the CBC. This test measures the various components of your blood. The main functions of blood are to carry oxygen, nutrients, and hormones to cells; protect against infection; remove waste products and toxins from the body. Blood is made up of many different types of cells. The three main components examined in a CBC test are Red Blood Cells (RBCs), Platelets, and White Blood Cells (WBCs). This may sound a little confusing, but it really is important for you to understand your blood counts. You should be able to know how you are doing. Following is an explanation of the function of each type of blood cell in the body, and the sign and symptoms you need to report to your doctor or the hospital medical staff.

WBC - **White blood cells (Leukocytes) fight infection.** There are three main types of WBCs. *Monocytes* defend the body against some bacteria such as tuberculosis. *Granulocytes* are divided into three cell types: neutrophils — which are the largest group of all white blood cells, eosinophils and basophils. *Neutrophils* fight infection by rapidly increasing in number, then surrounding and killing foreign substances. The neutrophils then quickly return to their original pre-infection numbers. They fight infections caused by most bacteria and fungi. *Eosinophils and basophils* also have infection-fighting roles. *Lymphocytes* are divided into two cell types which work with your immune system. *T-cells* attack viruses and cancer cells and control the function of other white cells. *B-cells* make and release antibodies. *Antibodies* are protein substances that coat infectious agents and mark them for removal from your body. When your WBC becomes lower than normal, you have an increased chance of developing an infection. You need to report to your doctor a temperature of over 100.5°, coughing and mucus production, or burning and pain when urinating.

RBC - **Red blood cells (Erthrocytes) contain hemoglobin, an iron-rich protein.** The hemoglobin picks up oxygen as it passes through the lungs. The oxygen is carried by the RBCs and given to the organs and tissues in the body. When the red blood cells are low in number, it is called anemia. When your RBC becomes low, you may feel weak, tired, or short of breath. Any of these symptoms needs to be reported to your medical team.

Platelets - **(Thrombocytes) are small disc-shaped cells that help control bleeding by helping blood clot.** Platelets prevent abnormal or excessive bleeding. When your platelet count becomes low, you may experience serious bruising and/or bleeding from a single cut or fall. Sometimes small reddish-purple spots, called petechiae can appear on one's body. The appearance of petechiae, unusual bleeding or bruising can be indicative of a low platelet count. Additionally, you need to report any bleeding from your nose or gums, blood in your urine or stool, or heavier or longer than normal menses.

There, now wasn't that educational!

CA125II

1 This blood test is given to detect ovarian and less commonly, breast cancer. This test reveals a protein released by tumors. It is not always reliable. The test is sensitive, not specific. In some patients their tumor doesn't produce the protein, or at least very little protein react. We have heard stories of patients with severe ovarian and low CA125 levels. Levels can be from under 10 to over 1000. It is not a great screening test, but it is good for following your cancer, especially if it was elevated before you were treated. If it does work in your case, a good rule-of-thumb is "anything under 35 is considered normal". Painless, it is a 1.

CEA (Carcinoembryonic Antigen)

1 Blood test that also measures levels of a protein. High is not good. This test is especially useful for colon cancer, and other gastrointestinal tract malignancies. Painless, it's a 1.

Bone Marrow Aspiration

9 This test is done to identify which type or types of cells are involved with suspected blood disease, and to monitor the status of a patient with blood disease (even after the patient is in remission). Bone marrow samples are usually obtained from the Iliac crests (hips). Less often, marrow is obtained from the sternum (breastbone). When a sample is taken from the hip, the doctor will ask you to lie on your side or stomach. The skin in the area is first cleansed and then numbed with a topical pain medication. A special needle is inserted through the skin and into the bone. A small amount of marrow is withdrawn through the syringe. The medication numbs the skin and tissue, but not the bone. The test usually takes only a few minutes, though it may seem longer. We definitely don't like this test, but it is so necessary that we say — just do it. Don't be afraid to ask for pain medication. It is a 9, maybe even a 10, but it's over quickly.

The first time I had this test, I decided that childbirth was much, much easier than a bone marrow aspiration (and I've done the childbirth thing four times). I remember walking out of the oncologist's office and telling my husband, "I'm never having another one of those! That hurt!" Little did I know. Since that time I have had many, many bone marrow aspirations, and although I still don't "enjoy" them, they are less painful than that first one. That is because, in addition to the topical anasthetic, my doctor gives me a mild sedative, intravenously, shortly before the procedure. It helps me relax, which reduces my anxiety and lowers the level of pain. — Shirley

---

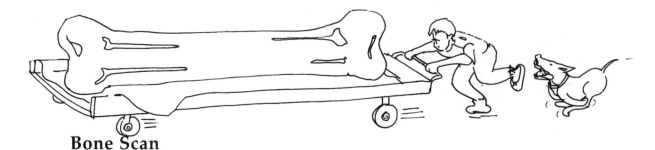

Bone Scan

1 This test is sometimes called a nuclear scan. A radioactive dye is injected into a vein. You idle away a few hours and return for the test. The radioactive fluid has traveled through your system. Do not worry; it is harmless and will leave your system quickly. The test itself consists of lying on a table. The scanner passes over and under you and relays images to a computer. They are looking for hot spots that appear to have activity. The test takes about an hour. Take a nap. It's a 1.

Brain Scan

1 A radioactive dye (isotope) is injected into a vein so that imaging of the brain can be done to detect any metastatic tumors. This one is also a 1.

Bronchoscopy

2-3 A test done with a thin flexible instrument (a lighted tube) inserted down the throat that permits the doctor to view the breathing passages. Unpleasant and uncomfortable, but not painful. We give it a 2 - 3, but only because of the gag factor.

CAT Scan

2 This test is also called a computed tomography or axial tomography scan. A series of x-rays taken in many directions is combined into one cross-sectional image creating detailed pictures of a particular area of your body. For scans of the gastro-intestinal area, and pelvic area, you will need to drink a couple of bottles of barium sulfate, a contrast to help see the intestines. (Lemon-flavored if you are lucky) and then a dye is injected into a vein to enhance the view capabilities of the x-rays. You may also have a barium enema. It's not too bad. The test only takes a few minutes. The dye is quickly flushed from your system. (Drink lots of water.) Depending on how you took your barium, by mouth or by enema, it can leave the body rather rapidly. Enemas may require a run to the bathroom. The barium can be a nuisance. We rate this as a 2.

Colonoscopy

3 A lighted fiber optic instrument is inserted in the rectum and fed up into the colon to look for problems. This test is a 3.

Colposcopy

3 Doctors have a magnified view of the vagina and cervix through an instrument called a colposcope. Tissues may be taken for biopsy. This test causes some bleeding and discomfort. We rate this a 3.

Conization

2   A cone-shaped tissue sample is removed from the cervix for viewing and pathology testing. This is usually done under general anesthesia. Discomfort is minimal. It is an outpatient surgery at the hospital. This is a 1 or 2.

Cystoscopy

3   The bladder is examined with a lighted fiber optic instrument inserted through the urethra, the tube that goes from the bladder to the outside of your body. Rather than painful, this test is "uncomfortable". To be safe, we rate this one a 3.

Digital Rectal Exam

1   Your physician inserts a finger into your rectum to examine the area for tumors. Weird, but painless. Rate it 1.

Dilatation and Curettage (D&C)

1-2   Tissue samples are removed from the uterus. The cervix is dilated and the endometrium is scraped with a curette (a small spoon-like instrument). You are put to sleep and you wake up a couple of hours later just fine. Take it easy after the procedure, but it is really only a 2. (In some cases, only a 1.)

Endoscopy

4-5   This is any one of a number of tests that uses a hollow, tube-like instrument to view and biopsy inaccessible areas of the body, such as the stomach, colon, bladder, lung or esophagus. Discomfort depends upon the area of the body being tested. From a 1 to possibly a 4 or 5.

Fluoroscopy

1   An x-ray procedure that makes it possible to see internal organs in motion. The fluoroscopy is painless. However, the positions you may be forced to assume during the procedure may cause some discomfort.

Intravenous Pyelogram of the Kidneys

1   A dye is injected into a vein and its clearance through the kidneys is tracked by x-ray. It may reveal blockages or tumors in the kidneys and/or connecting tubes. We give it a 1.

Laproscopy

2   A small cut is made in the abdomen. You will not feel this because you will be anesthetized and asleep. This test is done in the hospital (outpatient). A lighted camera instrument is inserted into the abdomen and it looks for cancer. A biopsy may be done at this time also. Small pieces of tissue will be removed and examined under a microscope to determine if cancer cells are present. You may be slightly sore at the site of the incision, but probably not. Maybe a 2.

Lumbar Puncture (Spinal Tap)

3 A long, fine needle is inserted into the spinal canal between the lumbar vertebrae and a small amount of spinal fluid is withdrawn for examination. The area around the puncture is anesthetized. You will have to lie on your side in a fetal position, or it may be done while you are sitting up and bending over a bedside table. You must remain perfectly still during the procedure. It sounds worse than it actually is. We give it a 3.

Lymphangiography

1 A dye is injected into the lymphatic system and x-rays are taken of the lymph vessels and nodes. We rate this a 1.

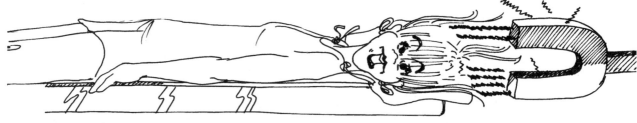

MRI (Magnetic Resonance Imaging)

1 A test that uses magnetic waves and a magnet linked to a computer to create images of certain targeted areas of the body. If you are claustrophobic, have someone go with you. The MRI technicians will put you on a flat bed, wheel you into a machine that looks similar to a large tumble dryer at the Laundromat and proceeds to make unusually loud noises for about 30 - 40 minutes. Have your companion rub your feet just to let you know that there is someone there. The technicians talk to you through a microphone. It is all very high-tech, but totally painless. Give it a 1.

Needle Biopsy (Fine Needle Biopsy)

1-5 A needle is inserted into an area suspicious of tumor to remove a small sample of tissue. This test is usually performed without anesthetic. The test will probably not take more than a couple of minutes, depending on what the doctor is looking for. The test can be just slightly uncomfortable to ouch. This rates 1-5.

Pap Smear (Pap Test)

1 Samples of cells are collected from the cervix via a small wooden spatula for microscopic examination. Not a particularly glamorous position to be in for a test, but it is painless. It's a 1.

Positron Emission Tomography (PET)

1 A radioactive injection of various tracer elements is traced through the organs of the body. This test provides excellent resolution. The test is usually looking for a specific type of cancer. It is done over different tracking periods. Some take 30 minutes, some longer. Not painful, give it a 1.

Radionuclide Scan

1 An exam that produces pictures of internal parts of the body. You are given an injection or an oral dose of radioactive material, and then a machine called a scanner measures the radioactivity of certain organs. Not painful, a 1.

Schiller Test

2 A diagnostic test in which iodine is applied to the cervix. Healthy cells stain, abnormal cells do not. Medium discomfort, 2.

Sigmoidoscopy

3 A procedure to examine the rectum and lower sigmoid colon to detect colorectal polyps and cancer. The physician visually inspects the area with a flexible, hollow, lighted tube. Samples of tissue or cells for closer examination can be collected through the tube. Some discomfort, but no pain. Can be about a 3, but only because it is unpleasant. Also called a proctosigmoidoscopy.

Transrectal Ultrasonography

3 A small transducer is inserted into the rectum. It allows the radiologist to make multiple biopsies. Pain level is 3. From what we hear, the anxiety level is usually worse than the test.

Ultrasound

1.5 Sound waves bounce off tissues and show echoes (sonograms) which are displayed on a computer screen. If it is a pelvic sonogram, you will have to drink a quart of water before the test to inflate your bladder. Do not drink ALL of it 30 minutes before; you will explode. Start slowly, about 30 minutes prior to the test. Don't let them scare you into thinking your bladder won't fill up in time. Believe us, a quart of water hits the old bladder pretty quickly. Get the last drop down a few minutes before your test. Don't tell the technicians we told you this. This definitely goes against their policy. Remember that you will have to check in at the hospital and wait your turn, and it is embarrassing when you start hopping around the waiting room with pee-pee panties. The rating for this test is 1.5, only because you may have to pee really badly with the pelvic sonogram. There is no other discomfort.

A breast sonogram is done by putting a gel on the breast and running a cold, flat instrument over the breast. It is usually performed as a diagnostic tool to look at tumors. This is a 1 for sure. Vaginal sonograms are often performed along with pelvic sonograms. A tubular thing is inserted in the vagina and it echoes back information. Other than feeling goofy while it is being done, there is no pain. We rate it a 1.

Upper Gastro-Intestinal Series (Upper G I)

1   A series of x-rays is taken of the esophagus, stomach and small intestine. You will drink a barium solution prior to the x-ray. Barium is a white, chalky substance that outlines the organs on the x-ray. This test is painless, but the barium is a little tough to swallow. We give it a 1.

X-ray (Roentgenography)

1   High-energy radiation is used in low doses to diagnose disease. This test involves standing in front of the x-ray machine or lying down on a table beneath the machine. The x-rays are painless, but sometimes the positions that you or your body parts are forced to assume can be uncomfortable. Generally, this is an easy 1.

We have only listed 35 tests in this chapter. There are, of course, many more tests in the doctors' diagnostic arsenals. When your doctor orders a test for you, ask questions and be persistent when requesting information on pain, discomfort and after-effects of the tests. DO NOT BE TIMID about asking for allowable medication to make the test more tolerable. We found that the nurses and technicians were especially helpful and forthright with us about pain and discomfort associated with certain tests and were very good about offering means of alleviating unnecessary distress. Talk with the medical staff PRIOR to the test so that if you need any medication, the doctor will have time to order it and you will be able to take the test with as little discomfort as possible.

 Note: Ask the test technician or physician administering your test to let you see the picture of the part of your body that they are testing. If you have a mental image of the area that they are treating, it is easier to visualize this area or organ getting healthy and cancer-free. It is hard to imagine a healthy, pink organ or cancer-free bone marrow if you don't know what it looks like. Visualization is an important tool in using your mind to help your body heal.

New tests are developed so rapidly that we may not have the latest information for you. These tests are current at the time of printing. If we have missed a few, that's great news. That means more diagnostic advances have occurred.

Take your worksheets along with you to the doctor
and to your tests. Use them.

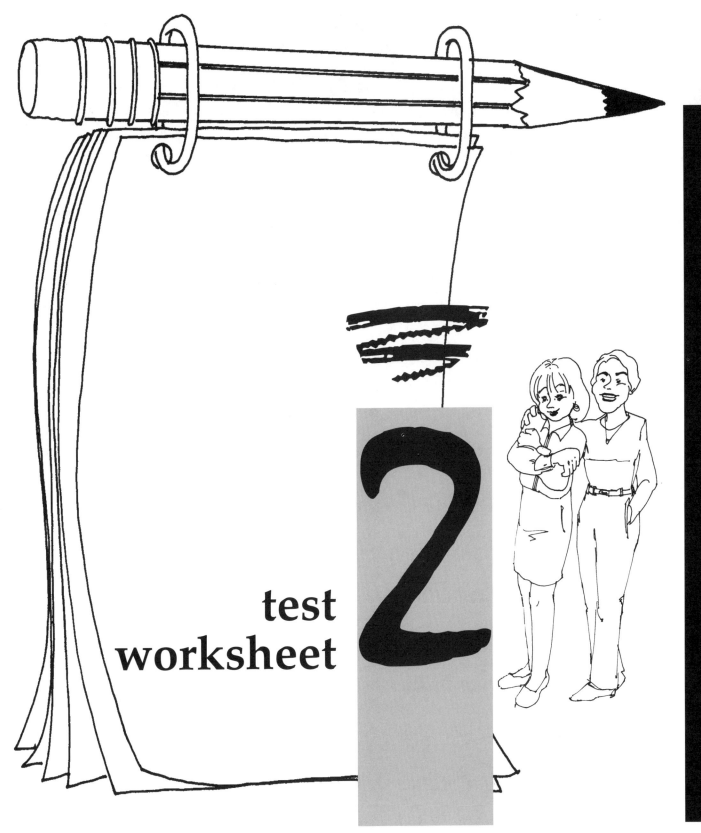

test
worksheet

2

test
worksheet

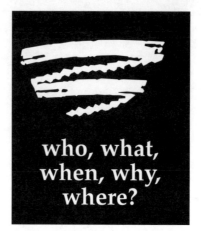

**who, what,
when, why,
where?**

Y ou may refuse any test. You do not have to submit to anything you are not completely comfortable with. But remember — if you do refuse a test, be sure of what you are doing. Your doctor may need the test information to treat you. Perhaps a different facility or technician would make you feel better about the procedure.

Do not let anyone manhandle or abuse you needlessly. You have enough to contend with. You need TLC. Make them give it to you.

You may stop any test if you feel something is wrong. Ask someone to (1) Explain what is happening. (2) Be more gentle, patient, understanding, or careful. Stand up for yourself. If you think something needs to be changed, *demand* it.

Name of the Test:

—⁓— What is the purpose of this test?
       A marker? (determining the level of your cancer, etc.)

       A detector? (determining if the cancer has spread)

       Understand why you are getting the test!

—⁓— Who will be performing this test?

—⁓— Explain the test completely and how it is performed?

〜 What can I expect during test?

〜 How long will it take?

〜 Where will it be done?   Home?   Office?   Hospital?

〜 Will I need to do anything beforehand to prepare for the test?

〜 Can a friend or family member be with me during the test? (*Unless there is x-ray or radiation, generally speaking you can have someone with you during most of your tests. If the staff says, "No", ask why. It may be they just don't want anyone in the way. Too bad. You can make the decision. If you want the comfort of a companion during the test, just ask them to make an exception. Stay firm in your conviction, and remember, you are in charge.*)

〜 Will there be any discomfort?

〜 Will I need pain medication or sedation? (*If you feel overly stressed, or expect the test to be painful, TELL YOUR DOCTOR. You don't need to endure any unnecessary pain or stress when medication can be administered to alleviate both. But your doctor must order this medication, usually ahead of time. The medical personnel administering the test are usually not able to provide medication for you. Whether you receive anything or not, try to calm yourself with your healing tapes or meditation. Remember: your mind can put you through real contortions. Don't let it make the test worse than it really is!*)

~ww~ How often will you do this test?

~ww~ What other tests will you run in conjunction with this one?

~ww~ How does one test relate to the other?

~ww~ How will I feel after the test? Are there any after-effects?

~ww~ How will the results of the test affect or apply to my treatment?

~ww~ When do we get the results and can I call you then?

~ww~ Can I get a copy of the results if I sign a release?

Strategy #3: Taking Command

Decide how, when, and where you will receive treatment. Treatment is defined by Webster's New Universal Unabridged Dictionary as: "medical or surgical care, especially a systematic course of this". To give you a broader definition, we wish to point out that treatment means two things: "the protocol designed to fight your disease and the way you are handled by your caregivers". Keep in mind that you are entitled to the best of both!

By now your chosen oncologist will have suggested a treatment plan for you. He has made his decision, but you haven't. You are about to embark on your next serious research project.

Your wellness may depend on the application of the latest cancer technology. You need to find out what that is. Your doctor may be right on top of things, but what if he is not? What if you are taking a harsher or less effective treatment than the large research facilities are offering?

To make a point here: one of the oncologists I interviewed told me my treatment for ovarian cancer would be a two-day stint in the hospital with an IV drip. What a drip-bag drag! My doctors in Cleveland had changed over to a three-hour drip sitting in a chair in front of the TV. Same medicine, different delivery. — Rose

Call other cancer facilities in and out of your area and ask the oncology departments about treatment options. Do your homework or you may suffer unnecessarily.

Your oncologist and all of the doctors you will see during your recovery have a great deal of influence not only on your care, but also on the quality of your life. Take time to understand the treatment planned for you. You must know what other options are available to you. If you need to get information on the latest treatments, call the National Cancer Institute or The American Cancer Society, check the Internet, or go to the library and research the most recently published medical journals. Check the appendix for sources of cancer information.

"The beginning of health is to know the disease."
- Cervantes, Don Quixote

Some cancer treatment is done on an outpatient basis; some requires hospitalization. Often, cancer treatment is a combination of both. You may have surgery in the hospital, followed by chemotherapy and/or radiation treatment as an outpatient. Or, your treatment may involve a prolonged hospital confinement. Either way, you are going to get to know your caregivers VERY WELL.

I spent the better (?) part of five months in the hospital for my leukemia treatment, and got to know my fellow patients and the excellent medical staff on a first-name, friendly basis. These people became my extended family during that time, as I was in essence "living" at the hospital. However, it was difficult to adjust to the prolonged confinement of hospitalization. I missed fresh air, freedom, and privacy. Even though we all like to be someplace where "everybody knows our name", the cancer ward at the hospital was not the site I visualized when I pictured being well known! — Shirley

---

Cancer treatment usually requires an extended involvement with medical personnel. With this in mind, we wish to note the following: you are paying for a service. The medical professionals treating you need to convince you that they can do the job and do it well. If they can't, take your body and your money somewhere else. Doctors and hospitals do not have to work hard to get patients. They come walking through the door every day. If they had to advertise by using satisfied customers, like most businesses do, then perhaps they would be more anxious to help you and make sure you leave happy and healthy.

Therefore, don't feel that you can't change your mind and your doctor. Doctors and other health professionals stay on their toes when they know they are dealing with an informed, assertive patient. If, however, your doctor is not receptive, find another doctor. If your hairdresser started giving you terrible haircuts (back when you had

hair, that is) you'd leave them in your dust. Don't get overly suspicious, but keep an eye on the care you are receiving. You and your doctors can get lazy and fall into a dangerous rut.

You may find after a certain amount of time a doctor can no longer be of help to you, or the quality of your care seems to be falling off. Talk to the doctor. This is your chance to make a change for the better and perhaps the next patient who comes along after you will benefit from your candor.

Don't make frivolous or emotional decisions, especially when you are taking medication, but don't stay with a physician you are unhappy with. If you decide to make a change, call and have your records sent to your new physician. Your former doctor will probably never confront you. His staff handles all the paperwork.

One of my physicians seemed very reserved and standoffish with me, never looking me in the eye when he spoke, standing at the foot of my hospital bed rather than next to it. I told him that his detachment made me feel like a "specimen", and that I really wanted him to remember that I was a person first, a patient second, and that I needed to be treated as "Shirley", and not "the leukemia patient in Room # whatever". I'm not a very assertive person, so I must have had some help here from the medications! Thankfully, he was receptive to my comments and made me feel quite comfortable about bringing the matter to his attention. I never felt that detachment from him again. — Shirley

---

Treatment and post-treatment usually involve some amount of prescription medication. If you are taking several different prescriptions, make a chart of the

> *"...medicine is a timeless art with a spiritual dimension and humanitarian purpose. Patients are not clients, doctors are not adversaries. Whatever the ups and downs of health care reforms, legal liability, economic pressures, changing forms of practice, and new science, doctors and patients alike must see this art as reality."*
> — Bernadine Healy, M.D.; A New Prescription for Women's Health

dosage and times to keep handy on the fridge or next to your bed. It will help any caregiver you may have, but more importantly, you can use it as a self-reminder to pop your pills. Keep a list of your medications in your wallet. It's a great safety precaution. Before you take any prescription medications, make sure you know why the doctor is prescribing them. You need a complete understanding of what is going to happen to your body while you are taking the drug. Do not see another doctor without getting the OK from your cancer treatment team. Make sure the new doctor has your complete medical history and that he sends all your records to your primary team doctor.

Drug and treatment interaction needs monitoring. Even over the counter drugs can be a problem. All medical personnel involved in your care need to be informed of any and all changes in your routine.

Try to use the same pharmacy for new and refill prescriptions. Get to know your pharmacist(s). Although personal, friendly service seems to be a thing of the past in the big chain drug stores, you can turn that around. Discuss your situation with the pharmacist. A good relationship may prevent script errors. We are not suggesting that they do make errors; rarely does that ever happen. But sometimes your pharmacist may catch a drug interaction that your doctor missed, especially if you have more than one physician prescribing. A good pharmacy will provide information on your medications with interaction and side effect details. Some drugs have very specific dosage regulations. You need to be informed.

What a lifesaver a good pharmacist can be! *Literally!*

You can refuse a prescription if you are worried about the effect it will have on you. It is best to discuss the drug with your doctor while you are face-to-face with him. However, if you don't, be sure to get all the pertinent info BEFORE you take the pill!

I had developed nerve damage in my hands from one of the chemotherapy drugs. The doctors had suggested an antidepressant with some neurotransmitter benefits. The drug also had a weight-gain side effect. No thanks; what else do you have? The next suggestion was a drug given to patients suffering from seizures. It had the side effect of drowsiness. I have to drive and function at work, and at least look awake. I chose not to take either of the drugs and just deal with the hand problem. You can make choices, too. — Rose

---

At the end of this chapter, we have provided a worksheet of questions to ask your doctor or pharmacist regarding prescribed medications. You will probably only have to use it a few times, and then you'll know the questions by heart!

Also, remember: don't keep old drugs. Dispose of them properly by flushing them down the toilet. Do not throw them out in the trash! Drugs may be found in the trash by animals and eaten, or scattered on the ground and picked up by a child!

The following information on treatments and side effects is current as of the writing of this book. New breakthroughs in treatment and clinical trials make headlines daily. Search the newspaper, Internet, medical journals. **Stay informed.**

Get any questions you have in your mind about your treatment answered completely. You must manage your care.

Stand up for yourself. Ask questions. Survive.

I sat in my treatment chair taking my chemo and chatted with a lovely lady next to me who was taking her second round of chemo after her second surgery for ovarian cancer. Her cancer had reoccurred in six months. The doctor had told her Taxol, which is one of the current drugs prescribed for ovarian cancer was not available. If she had known about Taxol and received treatment with it would it have made a difference? Maybe, maybe not, but I know I would have been really angry if I were her. Perhaps if she had inquired out of her area, she would have received the more current treatment. — Rose

Your cancer may be classified by "stage". This classification is made to determine the extent of the cancer in your body and the best treatment. Usually you will hear about Stages I, II, III or IV. This classification has to do with the spread of the cancer from its original site. The higher the stage number, the more advanced the disease. Your treatment will depend on the stage of your cancer.

The three most common types of treatment for cancer are **surgery**, **radiation** and **chemotherapy**. You may be given just one or a combination of these therapies. **Bone Marrow Transplantation (BMT)** is also being used more frequently to treat certain types of cancer, such as neuroblastoma, certain types of leukemia and lymphoma, as well as cancers of the breast, lung, ovary, germ cell tumors, multiple myeloma, certain childhood cancers and some primary brain tumors. It is a way to give higher doses of chemotherapy, such as the interlukens or interferons. Cancer may also be treated with biological treatments. New treatments are being developed in clinical trials. Gene therapy is a promising new treatment that is currently in trials.

Search the Internet to find more information. The National Cancer Institute at 1-800-4 CANCER has information on the latest treatments and trials available.

Surgery

Surgery may be performed to remove the cancer and surrounding tissues that are affected. This is why we suggested you find the very best surgical oncologist. Your life is in his hands. Your recovery period from surgery will vary depending on the amount of cutting and pasting done. Before you go into surgery blindly, use our worksheet to get all of the answers you need to be comfortable with the procedure. This surgery may increase your survival chances. Get more than one opinion on the specifics of the proposed surgical procedure.

My oncologist in Orlando prescribed four rounds of chemo and then debulking surgery to remove the tumor, then more chemo. This did not seem appropriate to me. My oncologist at the Cleveland Clinic suggested that the surgery be done first. I felt this would be less stressful to my system. Both procedures were acceptable current treatment; however, for me and my peace of mind, the latter was more appropriate. Trust your instincts. — Rose

---

You will be asked to go to the hospital for blood tests and x-rays before surgery. Be sure to take your insurance information with you. Also provide your doctor and the hospital with a complete list of medications, (including over-the-counter), that you are taking. Follow all of the instructions you have been given for the days before the surgery. Complications can arise from non-compliance.

Surgery can be very stressful to the mind as well as the body. Research has proven that stress can prolong hospital stays and impair the immune system's ability to heal. Information about the surgical procedures, what you can expect and how soon you can go home will take much of the fear out of the procedure. Hospitals often have pamphlets available through Patient Services or Admissions on what to do before surgery and what to expect after the nip and tuck.

Before you go into surgery, spend whatever pre-surgical days you have available powering up with nutritious foods: fruits, vegetables, juices, whole grains, vitamins. Give your body an extra boost to help it heal more quickly. Surgery will tax your system. Your body will begin to pull from many sources to sustain itself while under the distress caused by the surgery. Store up, like a squirrel for winter, the "nuts" your body needs to recuperate. Before changing your diet consult with your cancer team.

When you go to the hospital, bring something personal to put in your room. How about your most comfortable p.j.'s or nightgown? The ones the hospital provides are hindsighted and drafty. Bring your own slippers and robe. Don't worry about what they look like — they will definitely be more attractive than hospital issue, and ever so much more comfortable.

If you are in a semi-private room, ask to have the window side of the room. A sunny, peaceful view will be relaxing and help you heal. If you like to read, bring books or magazines. A tape player is great for listening to favorite tunes or your Dr. Bernie S. Siegel tapes. If you are having surgery as part of your treatment, have a friend or spouse set up your room for you before you get back from Recovery. It is nice to wake up to regular sights and sounds.

Laughter is an excellent healer.

Maintaining as much normalcy as possible is good for your emotional and mental health, which has a strong impact on your physical health! While recovering, turn on the television to watch comedies and have some good laughs. Laughter is an excellent healer. (Just don't split any stitches!) Make sure you are placed on a floor in the hospital that has other patients like yourself. Misery likes company? No, that is not the reason. Nurses who are used to caring for patients with similar surgeries and recoveries have helpful ideas to keep you comfortable. The nurses or aides will bathe you and will also give you back rubs if you ask. Remember: for what you are paying for that hospital room and all your $6 aspirins, you could be in a suite on the French Riviera. Try to get your money's worth out of the accommodations and staff. And before you leave, try to get a good supply of masks and gloves. You will need these in the future to protect yourself from germs!

Radiation Therapy

Radiation Therapy uses high-energy rays to damage and kill cancer cells. It is considered a localized treatment, as it targets tumors. Radiation can be delivered in two different forms, external and internal.

External Radiation is usually given in 5-day sessions for several weeks. This daily dose can be divided into smaller doses given more than once a day. Radiation can also be given for palliative care, to relieve symptoms. Intraoperative radiation is given at the time of surgery. The two days each week without treatment are used for rebuilding healthy cells that may be damaged by the treatments.

Internal Radiation is delivered by implants directly to the cancer-affected area. The implants may be temporary or permanent. You might make a Geiger counter jump for a few days, but before you leave the hospital you can sound the "all clear." You will not glow in the dark.

The three main side effects of radiation are *fatigue, skin irritation and loss of appetite.*

The extent to which they affect your daily life and overall feeling of wellness will depend on the duration and location of your treatment. Don't push yourself too hard. You may need to take daily activities a little easier too, like laying-off the long distance running, mountain climbing or heptathalon training!

Regular treatments can be time consuming. Arrange your appointments around work or other activities. Try to keep some normalcy in your daily routine. You may not want to eat; however, make sure to get something nutritious into your system. Try the liquid nutrient drinks. Chilled, with your eyes closed and distracted by loud noises, these drinks can simulate a milk shake. However, unlike regular milkshakes, they are packed with vitamins and minerals, not empty calories. Your body may be frantically

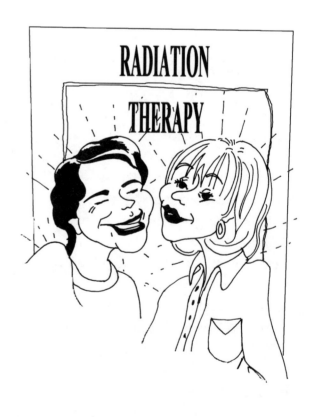

trying to rebuild precious blood cells and platelets to repair cells lost through treatment. You may want to increase your caloric intake. Be sure to eat fruits and vegetables and whole grains, if allowed. (Check with your doctor.) Give your body the fuel it needs to get the job done. Try eating when you are hungry, even if it's not at a scheduled meal. Listen to any cravings you may get. A desire for bananas may signal a need for potassium. A craving for spinach (honestly, I craved spinach! – Rose) may be your body's call for additional iron. We discuss this further in Chapter Six.

Even small meals during the day will help provide needed energy. Ask your doctors and nurses for their recommendations on ways to increase your appetite. Check with your doctor about what is appropriate for you. The Meals on Wheels program may help with prepared meals if you do not feel well enough to prepare food for yourself.

The American Cancer Society, your hospital, or your doctor may be able to help you locate these special types of service.

If you receive radiation treatment to the head or neck, take special care with your mouth, gums and teeth. You may experience stiffness, earaches from hardened wax, or a variety of skin changes. You may get mouth sores. A secret treatment (only known to

Treat yourself with care
**during and after the treatments.
Try these helpful hints
from the National Cancer
Institute:**

Get plenty of rest.
Good nutrition is a must.
Avoid wearing tight clothing
around the treatment area.
Treat your skin gently with mild
creams, soaps, etc.
Do not starch your clothes.
Do not rub or scrub treated skin.
Do not use adhesive tape
on treated skin.
Do not apply hot or cold packs
to treated skin; it is too sensitive.
Use an electric shaver.
Protect your skin from the sun.

about 5 million nurses) to relieve discomfort is "Magic Mouthwash". Actually, the nurses apply this name to any one of three or four mixtures. The mixture addresses a couple of obvious problems, cleans and numbs.

Obviously, this is *not* something you can or should mix up yourself, so ask for it. Check with your doctor before using *anything* on tender mouth tissue. And no alcohol in any preparation you use!

Another treatment used by oncology nurses is a five-day regimen of prescription throat lozenges.

Another nurse advocates the use of mints or other small candies or lozenges to keep healing saliva flowing in your mouth. Keeping the fluids going soothes the sores. The best care for mouth sores is the prophylactic approach — treating the mouth area before the sores have a chance to begin. Many hospitals have adopted this protocol to ease their patients' discomfort.

Radiation to the chest area may cause cough, fever and/or discolored mucous from coughing. If you are receiving treatment for breast cancer, try to go without a bra, especially an under-wire bra. It's sexy and very '60s. Retro is in now anyway!

You may experience a lump in your throat or swelling and redness in the breast. This may be from fluid retention. If you

Chemotherapy

Chemotherapy uses drugs to treat and kill cancer. Some drugs are more effective when given together which is called Combination Chemotherapy. Most drugs are administered through a vein or a muscle and some may be given by mouth. Chemotherapy drugs can be injected directly through the skin into a vein or can be delivered through a port or a catheter. It may be given directly into the cancerous area (intralesionally). Catheters can be placed in the Interperitoneal (abdominal) cavity, spinal fluid, bladder or liver. (This type of catheter is called intrathecal (IT), which means "in the spinal fluid".) There may be an internal or external pump attached. Your oncologist should advise you of your options.

Chemo is usually given in cycles. Your treatment may be administered once every 2 weeks, or maybe for a week, or even once a day. Perhaps it is only once a month. Your treatment schedule depends on your illness.

have implants placed in your breast or chest you may feel some stiffness or tenderness while they are in. Once removed, you may feel some of the side effects of external radiation.

If you receive radiation to the abdomen, you may experience upset stomach, nausea, and diarrhea. Nausea can be handled with an antiemetic. Ask your doctor for medications that are appropriate for you. You may do better on the treatments with an empty stomach. Try waiting a couple of hours after treatment to eat. If you get sick before your treatment, it's anticipation nausea. You need to try some relaxation techniques. The worry can make you feel worse than the treatment. Most symptoms fade within 10 to 12 months or sooner.

For treatment of my leukemia, chemotherapy was administered continually, via a Hickman catheter, for one full week. This course of treatment required an extensive hospital stay, and was repeated two more times. Obviously, with such a concentrated course of chemotherapy, the side effects can be quite pronounced and somewhat more severe than with other treatment regimens. And in some instances, normal procedure for dealing with side effects did not apply. I was not allowed to have fresh flowers in my room, to eat uncooked vegetables or fruits, or to use a regular toothbrush. I was given a little "sponge-on-a-stick" contraption which, once I got the hang of it, worked quite well! Clean teeth, no bleeding.

Everyone entering my room had to wash their hands, and when my blood counts were very low people entering my room needed to wear a mask to protect me from their germs. Flossing of teeth is a definite no-no, as well as shaving of body hair (No problem there. After week #3, I did not have any, anywhere, except for one recalcitrant hair on my right leg that must have been made out of stainless steel.) Actually, not having to shave should be considered a "good" side effect. The point I really want to emphasize here is that you need to be very sure that everyone entering your room abides by the rules. You need to put away your shyness and your natural submissive attitude toward those in the medical field and insist that everyone who visits or cares for you follows all the precautions." — Shirley

Keep an eye on your veins. Chemo can flatten out veins in your hands. If you have breast cancer and lymph nodes are removed from under your arm, you will have an increased chance for infections in that arm. Your lymph nodes strain infection. That means no blood is drawn from that arm, no blood pressure cuffs, etc. This limits you to the veins in your other arm. Keep an eye on your tolerance. Down the road, when you have recovered, you will still be checking back in with your oncologist for blood work. Sometimes it is hard to locate usable veins. Go on a Vampire Vein Hunt to identify some big, juicy veins that are popping out of the skin just waiting to be tapped. Be ready when the blood collectors call. Have the vampires search high and low for usable sites. These are your veins you are protecting.

By the time I was in for my 3rd go around with chemo treatments my veins had disappeared in my one good hand. The nurse was able to find a good vein on the side of my forearm just a couple of inches up from my wrist. It is amazing how many stick spots you really have (Once you have a mastectomy it is not recommended that you have a lot of blood drawn from your arm or take intravenous chemo if your lymph nodes have been removed.) Oh, by the way, IV needles don't have to hurt. — Rose

Because cancer cells grow quickly, cancer-killing drugs are designed to work rapidly. Chemo can effect rapidly growing healthy cells as well as the targeted cancer cells. Bone marrow, digestive tract, reproductive system, kidney, bladder, lungs, nervous system, and hair follicles can be damaged. That about covers all of the usual necessary working body parts, no? Chapter Six will give you more information on how to support your body systems during treatment.

A conquering hero, (that's you), wins the cancer battle! Be a victor, not a victim.

Bone Marrow Transplantation

A bone marrow transplant (BMT) is a procedure by which a patient's bone marrow is destroyed and then replaced with bone marrow from a donor. The donated marrow cells find their way to the bones and begin to reproduce and repopulate the patient's own marrow cavities and blood. Because a BMT is an involved procedure requiring four to six weeks of hospitalization and very strict care protocol, we are only going to touch on the basics in this book.

Chemotherapy and radiation treatment are used to treat cancer because cancer cells divide more rapidly than most other cells. However, in high doses, both these treatments can severely damage or destroy a person's bone marrow, leaving the patient without the means of producing needed blood cells.

In the case of chemotherapy treatment for leukemia, destroying the bone marrow is the purpose of the treatment, as the marrow is the source of the cancer. However, the intent of the therapy is to leave the patient with just enough marrow – hopefully, cancer-free marrow — to regenerate itself. It's a tricky procedure, which in my case worked out fine! However, to be safe, in 1995 I had a liter of my marrow "harvested" and stored (frozen) in case I need an autologous marrow transplant at some point in the future. — Shirley

---

When a patient's marrow has been severely damaged or destroyed, either intentionally or as a side effect of chemotherapy, a bone marrow transplant is necessary to replace the marrow. BMT's are divided into three groups according to where the marrow for transplantation comes from: autologous — the patient; syngeneic — an identical twin; allogeneic — a person other than the patient or an identical twin. Marrow transplantation can be done with either marrow, which has been removed from the donor's bone with a needle, or by peripheral blood stem cell transplantation (PBSCT), in which stem cells are removed from the patients circulating blood before

More than 10,000 bone marrow transplants are performed annually at approximately 200 BMT centers. The National Marrow Donor Program publishes a directory of these centers, the Transplant Center Access Directory. To obtain a copy of this excellent resource, write to:

Office of Patient Advocacy
3343 Broadway Street NE, Suite 400
Minneapolis, Minnesota 55413
or telephone 1-800-526-7809

There is no charge for this book. Also, the Oncology Nursing Society has a directory listing important information about 73 BMT centers.

treatment and then returned after treatment. PBSCT makes it possible for cancer patients to receive very high doses of chemotherapy and radiation therapy, as their marrow can be restored following those treatments.

BMTs are being done with increasing frequency and improving results. If your doctor suggests this treatment for you, once again you need to do your research. Just as when you are selecting an oncologist and a treatment center, the choice of where you have your transplant done, and by whom, is very important. You need to ask the same questions listed on the Oncologist Worksheet and the Hospital Worksheet.

Note: A BMT is a very serious procedure. Learn all you can about the treatment and the center that will be doing the procedure. You need to consider the following issues when choosing a BMT center:

⚊ With regards to the center itself, consider:

    The type of transplant to be performed

    The treatment plan (is it research or standard therapy?)

    The center's success rate for your disease

⚊ With regards to transplant team support, consider:

    BMT physicians' training

    Experience level of the nursing team

    Nurse to patient ratio

    Available psycho-social support

⚊ For financial support, consider:

    The cost of the transplant/treatment

    The center's experience in dealing with insurance companies

    Available financial services

⚊ For long-term follow-up, consider:

    The support the center will provide to your referring physician

    The center's availability to answer your questions

We realize that the information in this chapter may scare you, but this is not our intention. Remember that we are giving you information. Not everything applies to your circumstances.

Side Effects

The books and information you read about cancer tell you about the many possible side effects. You will probably not experience most of the ones listed. Nearly all can be treated and relieved during treatment. And, the good news is that almost always, the side effects subside after treatment ends. So you may have to deal with a few problems, but if they get rid of the cancer — just grin and bear them. There are clever ways to combat all of the side effects. Keep reading. We'll fill you in on some secrets.

All of the possible side effects will not hit you. You will probably only be plagued by one or two of them. Other than hair loss, all of them are treatable either through home remedies, such as resting when you are tired and taking additional vitamins (discussed in the Chapter Six), or prescription drugs to combat the symptoms directly.

Chemo Side Effects (ick!)

tiredness	weakness
vomiting	hair loss
anemia	bleeding
infections	diarrhea
constipation	mouth sores
flu-like symptoms	fluid retention
peripheral neuropathy	

(numbness and tingling in your fingers and toes)

When I heard I might get mouth sores, which I never did, I panicked. I was prone to canker sores and just knew it had to be worse than that. The oncology nurse at the doctor's office said to treat the sores like any mouth sore. "Don't worry — they can be managed." So don't panic — you can handle any of the side effects if you react to them promptly. Treat them immediately and do not be afraid to ask for medication. Keeping your body as comfortable and stress-free as possible is your goal during treatment. Stress is hard on the immune system. — Rose

---

Tips to Beat the (icks!)

According to the National Cancer Institute, which publishes excellent booklets on cancers and their treatment that are free to you by calling 1/800-4 CANCER, there are some easy things you can do to offset any discomfort you may experience during chemotherapy treatment.

- Avoid big meals, try 4 or 5 small ones.
- Drink liquids at least one hour before meals.
- Eat and drink slowly.
- Stay away from fatty foods and sweets.
- Eat foods at room temperature.
- Rest in a chair after meals; don't lie down for 2 hours.
- Avoid eating for 2 or 3 hours before treatments.
- Breathe deeply and slowly if you feel nauseated.
- Drink cool, clear, unsweetened fruit juices like apple or grape.
- Use an electric razor to avoid cuts.

The doctor will be able to tell you if your hair will fall out. If you will be losing your hair, get a short hair cut so that when it goes it is not quite as dramatic a change. That's the advice all professionals give. Even so, it is still traumatic when it falls out. It is dreadful to anticipate and when it actually happens you are frightened, mad, embarrassed and can't imagine how you will be able to stand looking that way for many months. Well, we are not going to kid you – it is awful! We both know first hand just how awful, but it is part of your cure, and will give you more years of life, so it must be dealt with and endured. It will get easier to bear. Do not be ashamed of your hairless head. It is your "Badge of Courage".

Take good care of your scalp and treat it gently! You may get the urge to tattoo it or use it as a geodesic pallet, but I recommend washable markers, only kidding. At least you can change patterns to match an outfit. — Rose

---

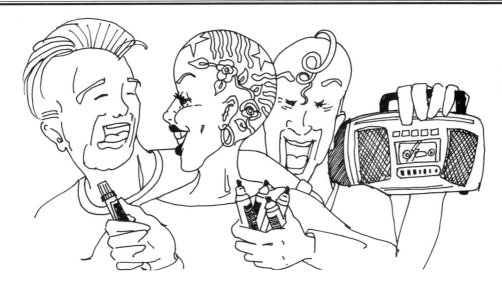

Chemotherapy may increase your risk of infection. Your white blood cells may be low. Without a normal white blood count you will have great difficulty fighting off an infection. Take care not to cut yourself. Avoid yard work, kitty litter pans, or any physical activity that could break the skin. If you do get a cut, your doctor may want you to be on antibiotics immediately. Call your oncologist and give him the details and let him decide what you need. Infection can become a deadly situation. See the next chapter for more information and precautions.

If you get sores in your mouth, treat them promptly. Topical treatment may give you some relief. Check with the nurses in your doctor's office; they quite often have the remedy. You might ask the medical staff for the "Magic Mouthwash" discussed in Chapter Three under Radiation Treatment. Other ideas include:

- Eat foods cold or at room temperature.
- Eat soft foods like ice creams (a fattening treat!), bananas, applesauce.
- Avoid acidic, spicy or rough foods.
- Use gravies, margarine, butter, and sauces to moisten food.
- Drink plenty of fluids.

How to handle:

Fluid Retention: Limit salt intake. Call your doctor and ask if you need a diuretic.

Diarrhea:

> Eat smaller quantities of food, avoiding high fiber foods.
> Avoid coffee and tea.
> Avoid raw, hard fruits and vegetables, esp: cabbage, beans, whole grain breads.
> Avoid roughage in general.
> Avoid alcohol and sweets.
> Avoid greasy or spicy foods.
> Avoid milk products.
> Drink plenty of mild clear fluids like water, clear broth, ginger ale.
> Eat potassium rich foods like bananas, potatoes, peach and apricot nectars.
> When you start to get better, eat foods high in potassium. You may have depleted your natural levels. Try potatoes, bananas, oranges, orange juice and low fat cottage cheese.

Constipation:

> Eat high fiber foods.
> Drink plenty of liquids.
> Exercise.

Peripheral Neuropathy:

> Peripheral neuropathy is sensory loss due to disease of one or more peripheral (outer parts of an organ or the body) nerves in the hands or feet; the syndrome can progress to muscular weakness and wasting.

This one I can speak on. This is the side effect that makes you the life of the party. Certain chemo drugs can cause temporary damage to nerve endings in the feet or hands. You then become a lot of fun to watch. You may feel tingling in your hands, feet, arms, and legs. The neuropathy may make it hard to button clothes, and you may act clumsy. My personal favorite was not having a real good grip. I could pick up a pencil or something light weight and a minute later it would go flying across the room as my hand moved only a couple of inches! (Told ya' you would be great party entertainment!) Just be careful in picking up hot drinks or anything you don't want to be wearing or literally sharing with a companion. It is irritating, but not awful. It can be rather slapstick sometimes. If you find the tingling to be bothersome or it wakes you up at night, sometimes shaking the arm or leg, as if it had fallen asleep, will help. — Rose

---

The neuropathy will continue for a few months after the treatments cease, but then should get better. It is our understanding that it is not permanent. Caution: advise your oncologist of the neuropathy as it progresses. It may be that he will want to adjust or stop treatments if it progresses too quickly.

Skin Problems:

How does the idea of dry, itchy skin sound? Peeling, cracking skin? Or for additional enjoyment, zits? Sound like a bad attack of winter-skin? You may experience a change in your skin during treatment. Treat the problem with mild lotions, creams and soaps. Cornstarch can be used as a dusting powder. Take shorter showers and baths. Use common sense in caring for your skin. The skin is trying its best to function normally even though the nutrients it needs are being depleted daily.

Sometimes skin can darken or redden along the vein where the drugs are injected. You can cover the area with make-up. It may be best to avoid direct exposure to the sun during treatment to protect your skin. Cover up if you are going to be outside for more than a few minutes.

"Radiation Recall" is a name given to a skin condition that may occur in an area previously treated with radiation. Reaction to the chemo drugs may cause a reddening in the area of radiation. Itching or burning may occur. Try pressing a cool compress on the affected areas. It is a short-term reaction and will disappear in a few hours or days.

Flu-like Symptoms:

Some cancer drugs may make you feel achy and miserable. All flu-like symptoms are possible: headache, fever, chills, poor appetite. These symptoms will all subside within a few hours or a few days, depending on the drug. Treat them as recommended by your oncologist.

Reproductive Problems:

Birth control should be practiced during treatment. The cancer drugs may have an effect on chromosomes. Pregnancy is not advisable. Break out the condoms.

Female reproductive organs can be effected by chemotherapy. Ovaries can produce less hormones or stop functioning completely during treatment. You may even feel some menopausal symptoms such as hot flashes, mood swings and depression. You may experience dryness or burning of vaginal tissues. Avoid oil-based lubricants like petroleum jelly. If you are having problems, your oncologist can prescribe a cream or suppository to relieve symptoms.

Insomnia:

If you are like us, the cancer experience makes sleeping difficult. Whether it is nerves or discomfort, even sleeping pills, which you can ask for, may have a difficult time putting you to sleep. Try the following ideas to relax and soothe your jangled nerves before going to bed.

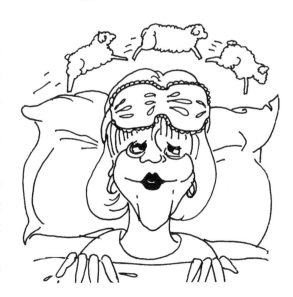

Don't go to bed until you are tired. It sounds silly, but many times you want to get additional rest and your body is just not ready. You'll waste a lot of time trying to force sleep.

Stay away from caffeinated beverages for up

to 8 hours before bedtime. That includes sodas, tea, coffee and trendy drinks. Read the label before you consume any beverage. You will be surprised how many contain caffeine.

Watch out for stimulants. Sugar is a big problem at bedtime. Unfortunately this means chocolate, ice cream, candy, cake, pies and all those really good comfort foods. These foods will put your body in high gear and make sleep difficult.

Check your medications with your pharmacist. Ask if any have stimulating or irritating side effects. You may need to change the time of day you take them. Vitamins should not be taken before bed. Some, like the B's, will energize your system. Others may cause stomach irritation especially since it has been hours since dinner.

Put yourself on a schedule. Pick a bedtime and stick to it. Regulate your system. Develop "before bed" rituals like having a cup of sleepy tea. There are many available on the market. Check your health food store or local supermarket. Try a warm bath. Set aside time for meditation or visualization on your own or with the help of a book or tapes.

Calm your mind. Somehow you must allow your thoughts to become peaceful. It is hard, especially when you are not feeling well. Just keep trying. It will happen. Create a formula that works for you and stick with it.

Nite nite!

I listen to meditation tapes by Dr. Andrew Weil. Even in the worst part of my treatments when you don't know if the chemo is working or not, the tapes let me drift off to another place where I am well and worry free. — Rose

---

Pain:

Pain: will you or won't you have some? The vote is to "not have it" of course. And you may not experience any pain. But if you do, do not hesitate to call for help. There are many ways to deal with it. We suggest using only what your oncologist recommends in over-the-counter medications. It is surprising how often common medications that you have taken all of your life can adversely affect your liver or kidneys. Be careful and check first. You will be going through a difficult time in your life; you may feel "not so pretty good". The last thing you need is to throw pain into the mix. If you need it, call for help and don't be afraid to complain to the doctor if you are uncomfortable. Why suffer? He is getting paid to get you through this situation.

If you are experiencing pain use the check list at the end of this chapter to determine the pain control program your doctor has planned.

If you are aware of all of the details you will be able to manage your pain symptoms and the stress they may bring with them. Stress can amplify pain symptoms.

When I was in the hospital, I had a doctor who came to my room and examined me every day. He asked about my discomfort and adjusted my medicine if I was in need of a change. He helped me make the decision to get off the medication pump which allowed me to self-administer my pain medication, and graduate to oral medication. He was called if I needed more medication and I felt good knowing that someone was tracking my situation. He was very responsive to my needs. You don't have to be in pain. — Rose

How to describe your pain to the doctor.

Give him the most detailed information you can. It will help him help you.

~~~ Remember when it started. Keep track of your symptoms.

~~~ Try to describe exactly were it hurts.

~~~ What does it feel like? Is it: stabbing, pinching, sharp, dull, achy, throbbing, sore?

~~~ How intense is it. On a scale of 1-10, 10 being awful, how does it feel?

~~~ What have you tried to relieve your pain? Have you taken any medications?

       If so, keep track of them so you can discuss them with your doctor.

~~~ Have you been able to relieve it at all?

Report to your oncologist:

Skin rashes

Frequent urination

Pressure to urinate

Chills

Loose bowels

White patches in the mouth (thrush)

Unusual vaginal discharge or bleeding

Pain or burning when you urinate

Reddish or bloody urine

Fever over 100°

Sweating

Sores in the mouth

Severe cough or cold

Redness, swelling, or tenderness around a wound, sore or catheter (Thrush)

Keep your Treatment Team informed of any changes you may be experiencing. You will feel better if they reassure you of the normalcy of your reactions and condition. You will feel in control and be more effectively managing your illness. If you experience any of the above symptoms during the weekend, when your doctors may not be available, write the symptoms down so that you can relate them to the doctor on Monday.

Things to do before treatment:

Have your teeth cleaned.

Have any essential dental work done.

Pick up a copy of Dr. Bernie S. Siegel's "Healing Tapes".
    Listen to them 3 or 4 times a day.

Make a list of medicines you are taking, over-the-counter
    drugs included .

Get control of yourself. If not, you may be your own
    worst enemy.

"Be optimistic. Optimists live through crisis, heal faster
    and have fewer complications. Optimists knew they
    were going home (from the hospital). Pessimists
    were afraid they weren't." *

Bernie S. Siegel, M.D., cancer surgeon at Yale University,
    said, "Positive emotions like love,
    acceptance and forgiveness stimulate
    the immune system."

* Fighting Disease, The Complete Guide to Natural Immune Powers; Ellen Michaud,
  Alice Feinstein and Editors of Prevention Magazine; Rodale Press, 1989.

Clinical Trials

Clinical trials in cancer research are done to evaluate new treatments and find better ways to help patients. Studies are done to analyze the effects of new drug combinations and of new and currently used drugs and therapies.

How do you know if you need to be involved? That confirmation may come from your cancer team, or it may be something you will have to determine on your own. There are many types of clinical trials. They can study many aspects of cancer including prevention, diagnosis, treatment, psychological problems, and pain control. They may focus on new areas of treatment such as biological therapy treatments.

Trials are usually managed in phases. The designated phases of clinical trial produce different types of information. You may be eligible for part or all of a trial depending on your particular cancer, age, or other variables. The federal government may support the trials, by private industry, or by grants.

Generally speaking, the ethical codes that govern doctors and the medical industry also cover clinical trials. However, if you do want to investigate the possibility of participating in a trial, do just that – *investigate the program*. Make sure that there are safeguards in place to protect you. For example, in a federally funded program, the Institutional Review Board (IRB) located at the institution conducting the test must check that the program is patient-safe.

Phase I - A new treatment is given to a small number of patients. The dosage is tested and the patients are watched for side effects. Although tested in the lab, this is the first exposure to humans. There may be a significant risk to the patient. Usually this phase is open to patients who have not responded to regular treatment.

Phase II - Studies are done to determine the effect of a treatment on various types of cancer. If the tumor is smaller and stays smaller the treatment is thought to be effective even if the response is as little as 20% of the patients.

Phase III - The new treatment is compared with standard treatment. Patients have a better chance of success at this stage. Larger numbers of patients are required for the study. Phase III looks for better quality of life and longer survival times.

Phase IV - The new treatment becomes part of standard treatment. It may be used in conjunction with existing therapies. This is obviously the best phase for successful results.

Clinical trial participation may seem frightening. As we have discussed previously, if you are informed about all aspects of the trial, and the risks and benefits to you, and of the part you play in the trial, you will take much of the fear out of the program. Remember that you are in charge. No one can make you stay in the trial if at any time you feel it is not in your best interest.

There are pluses and minuses to trials. If the trial is to test new treatments, you may or may not be successful. It is also possible to have short or long-term side effects from a new treatment. On the plus side, however, should it be successful, you will be one of the first patients to receive the benefit of the new therapy. You will also have helped other patients by advancing research on your type of cancer. Because a clinical trial is a new treatment, there is no way to be sure of the risks of the program. As usual, cancer forces you to make that important decision.

The National Cancer Institute publishes a pamphlet entitled, "What Clinical Trials Are All About". It will answer many of the questions you have about trials. They also have a computer file, called "Physicians Data Query (PDQ)" updated monthly listing over 1500 trials. It breaks the trials down by site of the cancer, such as breast, kidney, ovary, etc. It is available to you or your doctor and gives the names of hospitals, doctors, and trials offered all over the United States. The Cancer Information Service (CIS) will also answer questions at 1-800-4 CANCER. The staff will give you all the current clinical trial information and direct you to the research facilities conducting them.

The last time my ovarian cancer re-occurred, I decided to check into the new therapies in clinical trials. I called the National Cancer Institute. The staff member gave me all the info I needed on the gene therapy trials. I was given the name of the company manufacturing the product and the three hospitals conducting the studies. In one afternoon I spoke, not only to the trial coordinator at the gene producing company, but all three of the hospitals. Two of them agreed to take me into a trial. The particular trials had not done well on the ovarian participants. The hospitals were anxious to have another patient at a different stage of illness. The reason I chose not to enter the trial was that they were only in phase I. Trials are done in stages. Early on in the studies the results may not be confirmed. I chose standard treatment and decided to keep an eye on the trials to see how they were going. The point I am trying to make here is that you can be accepted into a clinical trial very quickly. Don't think they are hard to find or get accepted into. You may qualify. Explore your options. — Rose

We have a questionnaire at the end
of this chapter to use in reviewing
a clinical trial and
its relevance to you.

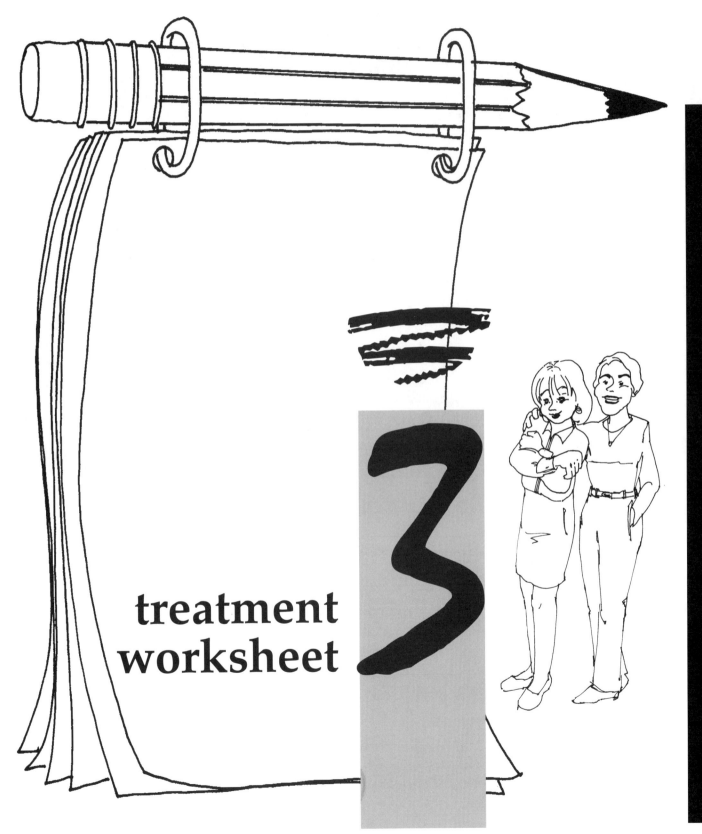

treatment
worksheet

3

treatment
worksheet

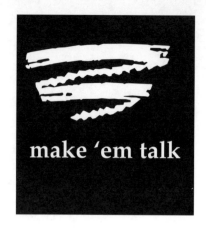

make 'em talk

What treatment plan do you suggest?

Surgery ___ Chemotherapy ___ Radiation ___ Other ___

~~~ Explain what you hope to achieve by this course of treatment?

Surgery:

~~~ Explain the entire procedure:

~~~ Where can I get more information on this?

~~~ What can I expect when I wake up? *(Pain, IV's, length of stay, etc.)*

~~~ What type of pain management will I have?

~~~ What do you hope to achieve?

~~~ What physical changes can I expect?

~~~ Where can I get information on adjusting to these changes?

~~~ Will I need additional treatment?   What kind?

~~~ What kind of discharge planning does the hospital have?

~~~ What will I need at home after surgery?   Medications/ homecare?

~~~ How soon will I be able to resume regular activities?

Chemo/Radiation:

⁓ How many treatments?

⁓ How long do they take?

⁓ How are they given?

⁓ Will I be receiving drugs?　　　　　Which ones?

⁓ Who will be giving them? What are their qualifications?

⁓ Do I take any by myself?

⁓ What if I miss a dose?

⁓ Can I take other medication?　　Here is what I take now:

⁓ Can I drink alcohol?

⁓ Can I take vitamins and herbs?

⁓ What over-the-counter drugs should I avoid?

~~~ Should I eat before a treatment?

~~~ Will I need a special diet?   If so, what kind?

~~~ Explain the treatment and the procedures?

~~~ How many team members will be monitoring my treatments?

~~~ How do I know that the treatments will be delivered properly?

~~~ What should I watch for to protect myself from a poorly
     administered treatment?

~~~ How safe are the treatments?

~~~ Will you give me pain or discomfort medication?

~~~ Will the treatments make me sick?   Nausea? Diarrhea? Other?

~~~ Will I gain or lose weight?

~m~ Will I need any additional treatments or other types of treatment during or after this treatment?

~m~ What risks are involved?

~m~ What other possible problems can develop from taking this treatment? *(Ex: other types of cancer, heart problems, bone marrow suppression, anemia?)*

~m~ Where do I receive the treatment?

~m~ What other types of treatments are offered for my type of cancer?

~m~ What is your projected goal? *(Shrink tumor, remove tumor, relieve symptoms, etc.)*

~m~ What are the possible side effects, in detail?

~m~ Are they temporary or permanent?

~~~ Do you have printed information that I may study to understand the proposed treatment?

~~~ How many other patients that you have treated have been successful in stabilizing their conditions with this type of treatment?

~~~ What can I do to minimize the effects of the treatments? *(If he does not know, ask his nurse or check with the hospital oncology department or other cancer resources.)*

~~~ How will you measure the effectiveness of the treatments?

~~~ What tests will you be using to monitor my progress?

~~~ Will I have to go into the hospital?

~~~ How much will the treatments cost?

~~~ Can you accept only what my insurance company pays? *(The costs can be astronomical.)*

~~~ Am I eligible for clinical trials?

prescription worksheet

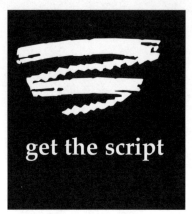

get the script

〰 Exactly what does the medication do?

〰 Do I really need to take it or is it optional?

〰 What side effects and drug interactions do I have to be aware of?

〰 Are there any foods that I need to avoid while taking this medication?

〰 Exactly what is the dosage and how do I take it?

〰 Do I have to take the pills: With water?   With milk?

On an empty stomach or a full stomach?

Before meals or after meals?   AM or PM?

During the night, or at intervals during the day only?

〰 How soon will I see results?

~~~ What if I don't see results in that time period?

~~~ What over-the-counter drugs should I stay away from?

~~~ Can I use the generic brand (if available)?

clinical
trials
worksheet

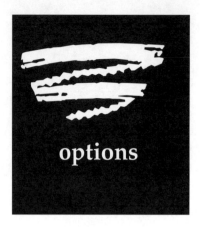

options

〜 What is the purpose of this study?

〜 What phase are you in? Describe the phase breakdown and the purpose of each phase.

〜 What does the study involve?

　　　What kind of tests and treatments?

　　　How is each of them done?

〜 What could happen to my cancer with this new treatment? Without this treatment?

〜 How is this study different from standard treatment?

〜 How long does the trial last?

~~~ Do I have to be in the hospital, or can I come for out-patient visits?

~~~ Who is in charge of the study?

~~~ Who will be reviewing the results?

~~~ If the results are successful, will I have access to the treatment after the study?

~~~ If I am harmed by the study, will there be care available to me?

Will I have to pay for the care?

~~~ Will there be a cost to me to participate in the study?

~~~ Am I obligated to stay in the program if I am not comfortable with it?

~~~ What type of long term follow-up is offered?

~~~ Will I be able to continue normal daily activities?

~~~ What physical and emotional changes should I expect?

pain
management
worksheet

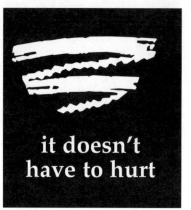

**it doesn't
have to hurt**

〜 Will I experience pain from:

       Treatment?

       The cancer itself?

       Surgery?

〜 Who will help me control it:

       You?

       Hospital?

       Staff?

〜 In the hospital, is there a pain management physician assigned to me?

〜 How can I recognize the difference between everyday to-be-expected pain and something more serious?

〜 Where do I go and who do I call in an emergency?

〜 How do I really get through to you in an emergency? What do I tell your office or answering service?

〜 Do you know of any non-medication pain management techniques?

〜 Does the hospital have any pain management programs that might be helpful?

Strategy #4: Protect Your Body from Infection

Cancer disrupts your life - this is the understatement of the century! There is no way around that fact. But you can minimize the disruption. Any changes you have to make in your routine can be controlled. Your conscious decisions will regulate the quality of your daily life. While you are undergoing treatment, you may not be feeling like your old self, and rightfully so. Some of the standard cancer treatments, such as chemotherapy and radiation, destroy healthy cells in addition to the cancer cells. Your immune system is effected, and has to work very hard to keep you as healthy as possible. All of your other organs will be affected by the treatment, too, and working a little harder than usual. You need to be aware of the stress your body is under, and do all you can to make its load a little lighter. Taking sensible precautions during and after treatment will help you maintain a healthier body and the bonus is you'll feel better!

Many doctors will take the time to tell you how to protect yourself during and after treatment. Some will not. Oncologists are often very busy and expect you to "just know". Your healthy cells may be suffering while your cancer cells are being zapped. If this is the case, it is your duty to give the healthy ones a fighting chance. Ask the oncology nurses in your doctor's office or in the hospital if they have any printed information on how to protect yourself from the germs that are waiting for you at every turn in the road. The National Cancer Institute and the American Cancer Society often have pamphlets right in the doctor's office. The nurses themselves are an incredible source of information and may have some tricks-of-the-trade to share with you. If you really want to know how to get through this situation, you need to ask questions yourself, take charge, and, as we keep emphasizing, be informed.

My oncologist prescribed chemotherapy for treatment of my breast cancer. I was determined to continue my normal activities. He offered no special information on what to take to make this procedure as easy as possible on my "insides". I asked his nurse, and she said to drink water, more water, and then just to be sure, drink some more water. I walked around for the next nine months with a large bottle of spring water in my hand. It really helped to keep the stomach problems away. I think it may have helped prevent other irritating side effects, as well. Maybe I only thought it did, but it worked for me. It was good advice! — Rose

Germm Warfare

Treatment for cancer usually lowers your immune system response. You have to take special care of yourself, and it is essential to protect yourself from the bacteria and germs that lurk EVERYWHERE. Be careful. Think about everything you touch. Unconsciously, we put our hands to our mouths and eyes. Many germs enter the body this way. Once you stop and think about the world of germs that we face every day, you may begin to develop a white glove phobia. Don't go to extremes, but keep your hands clean. Wash them with soap and water OFTEN.

The following list of Do's and Don'ts will help you make it through the treatments and return to a healthier person after your regimen is over. We repeat ourselves at times, but that is only to reiterate important points, and because at our age sometimes we tend to repeat ourselves!

Observe the Following Mandatory Rules of Self - Preservation:
Do:

Listen to your body. It will tell you if it needs help. Answer its call.

Laugh. Often. Laughter is incredibly good medicine.

Question every procedure, medication, and instruction. Gain a full understanding before you proceed.

Check with your pharmacist and/or doctor regarding all prescriptions and over-the-counter drugs. Side effects and interactions can be dangerous to you.

Carry a card with you at all times that lists all the drugs (prescription and over-the-counter) and vitamins that you are taking, along with the dosage amounts. Keep the card with your medical insurance card(s) and it will always be handy when you need the information.

Wash your hands, including the back of your hands, in warm soap and water after:
Shaking hands
Touching other people
Handling pets
Putting dirty clothes into the washer
Working in the yard - dirt contains germs, mold and fungi.
Taking out the trash
Handling public telephones

Touching doors, doorknobs, and handrails in public buildings

Touching anything in a public restroom! (See "Public Germs" (next page) for detailed advice on how to get in and out of a public restroom SAFELY!)

Stay away from recently immunized children, (measles, polio, etc.) You might contract the disease and have difficulty fighting it off. (Not all vaccines are live viruses; just be careful.)

Avoid friends or family or strangers with flu or cold symptoms.

Wear shoes to protect your feet against cuts and scrapes.

Keep kitchen counter tops clean with disinfectant soap and water.

Keep your nose moist with saline solution sprays. Bacteria can enter through cracks in the membranes.

Use lip balms to keep cracks from forming on your lips to avoid bacteria entering the body.

Use tissue instead of handkerchiefs. Don't carry around a dirty hanky.

Close the lid on the toilet to avoid airborne bacteria. In a public washroom, wear a mask if you can.

Apply creams to keep skin soft and prevent drying and cracking.

Wear sunscreen and protective clothing to prevent sunburn.

Wear a hat or scarf to protect your face and head from too much sun. This is not a good time to get sunburn.

Exercise to the best of your ability, even if it means only walking a short distance.

Try to maintain regular daily activities. The normalcy is good for your mental health.

Eat a balanced diet. Good nutrition aids in your recovery and helps rebuild damaged tissues and fight infections.

Drink lots of water and other fluids. Clear fluids are easiest on your body.

Ask for help when you need it. Don't be afraid or ashamed. We all need help some times! Most people will reach out to help you. A kind gesture will mean a lot to you. When you are well, do the same for others.

Stand up for yourself if you feel you are not being listened to or cared for properly.

Reach out for emotional support through groups or fellow patients.

Don't:

- ⊘ Be afraid to ask your doctor: "Why?"
- ⊘ Be afraid of your doctor!
- ⊘ Be afraid to question your doctors whenever you need an answer. Feel free to be brought up-to-date on your condition. (You are paying them - not the other way around!)
- ⊘ Take any medication, including aspirin, without checking with your oncologist. (Even over-the-counter medications you may have been taking for years.)

- ⊘ Use drugs containing ibuprofen unless approved by your doctor.
- ⊘ Let depression or anxiety get the best of you. If you are having trouble coping, ask for help. Depression and anxiety are common side effects of dealing with cancer, and can be treated.
- ⊘ Enter a teenager's bedroom without protection (mask, gloves, disinfectant). *Humor!*
- ⊘ Be afraid to warn family and friends to stay away when they are sick.
- ⊘ Share towels, wash clothes, toothbrushes, razors, or other personal items.
- ⊘ Be afraid to tell someone you are sick and need special attention.
- ⊘ Forget to laugh! Often!

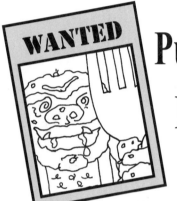

Public Germs

Do:

Rinse and wipe silverware in restaurants. Use your napkin and water from your water glass. Using a pre-packaged alcohol wipe is even better. Surprisingly, there is no alcohol taste left on the utensils!

Wear a surgical mask in crowded situations such as malls, church, parties, etc.

Take the following precautions when forced to use a public restroom:

Public restrooms require extra special care. Never touch the door handles, the taps, or the flush handle with your bare hands! If you are limber enough, use your foot to depress the flush handle. If not, use some toilet paper in your hand to depress the flush handle and then throw the paper into the toilet. Get paper towels and put them under your arm, wash with soap and water, wipe your hands and then turn off the tap with the towel.

Dispose of the used towel(s) OUTSIDE the restroom. You will need the towel to open the door when you leave. Not everyone has the same high-level personal hygiene habits that you do, and the germs that are living in profusion on the entry/exit door handles of public restrooms are too disgusting to consider. Not everyone washes their hands carefully, if at all, after using the toilet, and knowing where those hands have just been, one shudders to think of what might be on that door handle. Considering the enormous number of germs present in public restrooms, it is an excellent idea to request that all your family members and friends abide by the above precautions. Everyone will benefit, and these are good habits to form.

Don't:

- ⊘ Eat from a restaurant or grocery market salad bar.
- ⊘ Drink out of a public water fountain.
- ⊘ Take candy, food, toothpicks or any item that is in a communal container.
- ⊘ Drink or eat from anyone's cup, glass or plate.

Stay Healthy - Disinfect!

- ⊘ Eat food at a restaurant or roadside stand that looks even slightly unsanitary.
- ⊘ Swim in community pools or hot tubs.
- ⊘ Handle pets that are ill.

Private Germs

Do:

Let someone else clean out all the unidentifiable growths in your refrigerator. It may well be a form of penicillin, but not the form you need!

Get someone else to clean the bathroom. You don't need that kind of close contact with bacteria, but you do need a clean bathroom.

Have someone clean the heating system and air/conditioning system in your home, while you are NOT there. Nasty things lurk in the vents, filters, etc. Change the filters often.

Wash fruits and vegetables with soap and water, or vegetable wash (available at health food stores), to dissolve and remove waxes and pesticides.

Cook all foods completely. You do not want to get salmonella or E Coli from eggs or meat.

Rinse all meat and seafood before cooking it. Other people have been handling it!

Rinse your toothbrush (in alcohol or boiling water) and keep it in a clean, dry place to prevent unnecessary germ growth. Note: Use a soft toothbrush.

If your blood counts are low, check with your doctor regarding the safety of flossing. *(Bleeding can be a problem, and any cut in the gums will encourage infection.)*

Avoid mouthwashes that contain salt or alcohol.

Use lubricants to treat vaginal dryness. (But no lubricants that contain petroleum products!)

Consult your doctor regarding birth control methods during treatment.

Use condoms to avoid infection.

Bathe, shower or cleanse yourself daily. Soap and water are a great defense against bacteria. Use warm, not hot, water and towel dry gently.

Use lotions if your skin becomes dry. Cracked, itchy skin is not just uncomfortable, it is an infection risk.

Clean cuts and scratches immediately with soap and water and apply antiseptic.

Enjoy your family pet(s), but decrease close exposure.

Don't:

- ⊘ Drink alcohol. It is hard on your already over-worked liver and kidneys.
- ⊘ Use suppositories. They may cause rectal bleeding.
- ⊘ Use a razor. Use an electric shaver to avoid cuts.
- ⊘ Use tampons. They could cause infection.
- ⊘ Wear contact lenses without checking with your doctor.
- ⊘ Use hair removal products.
- ⊘ Cut your cuticles.
- ⊘ Squeeze pimples.
- ⊘ Get any immunization shots without checking with your oncologist.
- ⊘ Clean litter boxes, animal cages, or your yard of animal waste (a.k.a. pet poop).
- ⊘ Use an IUD without your oncologist's approval.
- ⊘ Use a diaphragm until your blood counts are normal.
- ⊘ Have sex with partners who have had unprotected sex or a history of sexually transmitted disease.
- ⊘ Use anyone else's bar of soap - too many germs!
- ⊘ Be afraid to speak up! If, because of your low blood counts, you are under "isolation", either while in the hospital or at home, don't be shy about insisting that all visitors abide by the rules. They should wear masks and gloves while in the room with you, or at the very least, wash their hands with soap and water before coming in contact with you or anything you use.

Fatigue
Or
Are You Too Pooped to Pop?

One of the most common complaints of cancer treatment is fatigue. You may feel tired, weak, irritable, or unable to concentrate. Other symptoms may include loss of appetite and withdrawal from social activities. Anemia, cancer treatment, chronic illness, medications, poor diet and a lack of, or too much rest can cause fatigue. We have dragged around ourselves and have learned a few fatigue fighters.

Here's what we found:

✘ Ask for help if you need it, don't try to do more than you should.

✘ Drink water, and more water, 8-10 glasses of non-caffeine fluids daily.

✘ Maintain a well balanced diet with focus on low fat foods.

✘ Eat small meals throughout the day, instead of 3 big ones.

✘ Get out of your chair and move around, a little light exercise might help.

✘ Limit your naps to 30-45 minutes at a time.

✘ Maintain a regular sleep schedule, get up at the same time each day.

✘ Stay in touch with your doctor and advise him of your status.

You may want to keep a record of your symptoms and your activity ability. Then when discussing it with your doctor you can tell him specifics rather than, "I have just been feeling tired the last few days." Ask your doctor for help. There are medications available to relieve some of the symptoms. You don't have to be miserable during treatment.

You may feel tired for a while after completing your treatment. Your body will need time to recuperate. Bring balance back into your life with meditation, good nutrition and exercise. Like us, you will get back to normal energy levels with time and some TLC.

While I was in the hospital for my induction chemotherapy, I developed pneumonia. The infection came at the point at which my blood counts were at their lowest, and I am here today mainly because I had an excellent, persistent and determined team of doctors, including the all-important specialist in infectious disease. My life was dependent on his ability to find the right antibiotic. This was not a fun time for any of us. But the point I wish to make is that, in retrospect, I realize that I was careless in following the "Do's and Don'ts" for immune-suppressed patients. I did not speak up when people entered my hospital room without the mandatory surgical mask. Nor did I insist that every visitor wash their hands immediately upon entering my room, even though that rule was posted on my door alongside the box of mandatory masks. I may not have contracted the pneumonia from a visitor — it may have just been floating around in the hospital, a rather common place for it to be — but still, I took a risk with my life by not being assertive about my own well being. Don't make the same mistake. — Shirley

Special Note of Importance:

If you have a Hickman catheter, don't shower. Take sponge baths and keep the port area meticulously dry. Most medical personnel will tell you that showering while having the Hickman in your chest is all right. We don't agree. This is a non-medical opinion – always check with your cancer team.

I had a Hickman catheter implanted in my chest for 7 months. (Actually, I had two. The first one fell out. Occasionally this happens. It was no big deal, just scared me a little and required the surgical implant of a new one.) The doctor told me that it was perfectly all right to shower with the Hickman in. But a fellow patient, a good friend who did some research on the matter, and a nurse told me that they did not agree. The Hickman port is a main access to the heart, and therefore a direct entrance for germs. I thought about the dirty, soapy water that would be running passed (and into) the catheter entry point during the process of showering, and opted not to take the risk. I stand by that decision 100%! I did not get one single infection in my Hickman, and I don't know many other patients who can make that claim. With the absence of body hair, and my rather limited physical activity level during treatment, I did not find that taking sponge baths compromised my hygiene in any way. I was still sweet and clean; well, clean anyway. — Shirley

Another Special Note of Importance:

If you have had a mastectomy, take special care to protect against Lymphedema. Lymphedema is the buildup of lymph fluids in subcutaneous tissues. This can occur in the arm after lymph node removal, a fairly common procedure accompanying mastectomy. If infection occurs in the arm, it can become swollen, heavy, tight and uncomfortable. Other problems include immobility and unpleasant appearance. It can be difficult to return the arm to normal appearance and function. You can help avoid problems by:

✘ Covering up in the sun. Avoid sunburn.
✘ Being careful not to cut, scrape the skin.
✘ Wearing protective clothing to protect against insect bites and rashes.
✘ Not cutting your cuticles.
✘ NEVER having blood pressure taken in that arm!

Baby the arm and guard against abuse. This is not an excuse to get lazy. In fact, exercise is great for circulation. Just keep an eye on your physical environment and your arm should be fine. But if you do get a cut or scrape, disinfect it immediately. Clean the wound and bandage if needed. Change the bandage frequently. At the first sign of a problem, call your doctor.

My arm has functioned in my "cuts and scrapes" world for six years. It has been in great shape. However, I have been able to use the "big arm" thing for sympathy and as a cop-out for my flabby upper arms. "Oh, I'm not able to do too much with the arm! (or arms)," depending on how hard I am trying to defend the flapping flesh. Protect your arm(s). It's not a lot of work, but the alternative IS. — Rose

"Words are, of course, the most powerful drug used by mankind."
- Rudyard Kipling

Don't let hope get trampled by careless comments or diagnostic mumbo jumbo. You are unique and so is your illness. No one, especially not the doctors, can predict your future. The power to heal is within you. Don't be upset and disrupt your natural abilities to fight your disease. Hope will improve your quality of life. Never give it up no matter what is said to you — Rose.

Traveling Germs

Although the aforementioned rules for protecting yourself during your cancer treatment obviously apply while you are traveling, there are some extra precautions you need to take. If we repeat some of the previous "Do's and Don'ts", it is just to be sure that you understand the importance of protecting yourself against the added germ-laden climate that you face in a travel environment.

Airplanes

Most airlines recycle air during flights. All of the coughing and sneezing done by hundreds of people on your flight is blown back on you while you head off into the wild blue yonder. We traveled with a surgical mask and gloves. We purchased ours at a medical supply store, generally located near the hospital. If you can not find a medical supply store, ask the home health department in the hospital for a list of area stores; or pick up painting masks at a home improvement store. Those work almost as well and usually cost a little less.

If you have a depressed immune system or are recovering from surgery, wear a mask and gloves in any circumstance where you are not in control of the people around you. Even though you will look like an alien, it will help keep the germs out of your system.

On one of my flights, a flight attendant stopped by my seat and said she wished she could wear a mask. She said she was sick all the time! — Rose

If you are wearing the mask, you can board when they call for first class passengers or anyone needing special assistance, allowing you to board the plane early. This is helpful when trying to find overhead space without being shoved and pushed by other passengers and makes it easier to get to your seat comfortably.

When you have to connect to another flight, don't walk between gates. At the time that you make your reservation, or upon arrival at the airport, ask for a wheelchair or a tram to meet you at your flight. As you know, your flight is always assigned to the remotest gate in the terminal. Swallow your pride and ride. You will enjoy the pampering.

Ask for aisle seating. It affords the most leg room and is an easy exit. If you really want to stretch out ask for the bulkhead seat. Don't volunteer for the exit rows. On many airplanes the exit row seats do not recline. And, you may not be strong enough to open the door in an emergency.

If you are traveling alone, do not try to carry your own bags. At baggage claim or in the terminal, the skycaps will be happy to help you and take you to your gate, baggage claim or to ground transportation. They work on tips and at about a dollar per bag. It is a physical relief well worth the cost.

Carry a small thermal lunch bag with you on long flights. It is great for carrying fresh fruits and snacks. Many of the airlines only provide liquid refreshments. You can carry bottled water. Water may be pumped on board from trucks and stored in the plane's holding tanks. One can only imagine what is growing on the bottom of those tanks. Ice may be made from the same water source. You want to avoid the bacteria. Although you obviously have to take your mask off to eat, get it back on as soon as you are finished. Some planes have room to store cold items for you, but don't count on it. If you eat the airline food, remember to wipe off any utensils that are not sani-packed. Actually, to be safe — wipe off those too.

"Rose and Shirley's Never Get Cooties Rules"

✘ Wash your hands with soap and more soap and warm water.

✘ Wipe with paper towels you have pulled prior to washing.

✘ Wipe, and then, (now here is the tricky part), use the towels to push the flush button and open the slider on the door. Hold the door open with your elbow and then throw the towel away. You do not have to touch anything in the restroom with your clean hands!

When using the restrooms on board, use the following **"Rose and Shirley's Never Get Cooties Rules"**, and the rules for using public restrooms under the heading **Public Germs.**

✘ Wash your hands with soap and more soap and warm water.
✘ Wipe with paper towels you have pulled prior to washing.
✘ Wipe, and then, (now here is the tricky part), use the towels to push the flush button and open the slider on the door. Hold the door open with your elbow and then throw the towel away. You do not have to touch anything in the restroom with your clean hands!

Cruise Ships and Trains

Masks and gloves – use them. Abide by the Public Germs and Never Get Cooties Rules! Wipe off all silverware! As with airplane travel, don't be afraid to ask for assistance in getting to and from the train and the station.

Automobiles

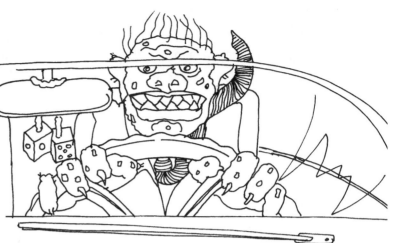

If the air-conditioner or the heater in the car is on, wear your mask. Germs breed in both the heater and the A/C. If anyone else in the car is coughing, sneezing, or discharging germs in any way, wear your mask. If you are riding in your own car, you can control the cleanliness of your environment. Be sure your car is as clean as possible. However, when traveling in someone else's vehicle, it is wise to take a few extra precautions, such as wearing gloves. Don't worry about offending anyone. Better that someone be slightly insulted by the connotation that your precautions imply, than that you get sick. A suppressed immune system is not something to fool around with. This is your health and your life at stake. Offending someone is better than fighting for your life because you were careless and too concerned about hurting someone's feelings.

My husband kept our car immaculate while I was undergoing my chemotherapy. Our car smelled positively antiseptic, and as long as the heater or A/C was not on, I could ride mask- and glove-free. However, I did offend an acquaintance who offered to drive me to the store during one of my between-treatment interludes at home. Her car was quite "unsanitary", and I was afraid I would pick up bacteria from the door handles, or inhale germs from all the trash on the floor, so I wore my gloves and mask. She was insulted. After I explained how meticulous I had to be with my health, she eventually understood. Nevertheless, even if she had been permanently hurt by my actions, I still would not have done anything differently. I like living. — Shirley

Hot Air Balloons

No problems here – just have a good time!

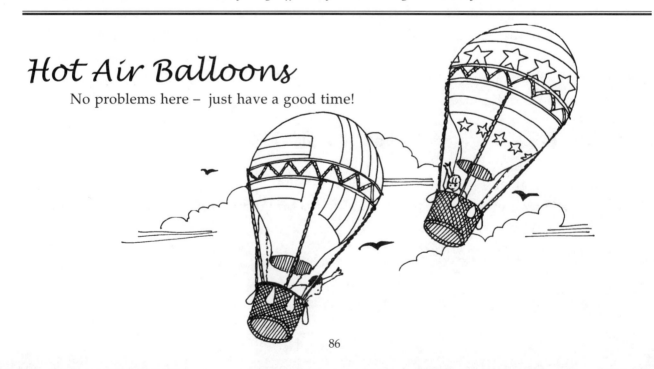

We hope we haven't frightened or overwhelmed you with all the "Do's and Don'ts" in this chapter. These must seem like a lot of unnecessary or laborious precautions. They may very well be, in some cases. But keeping up on the "Do's and Don'ts" can prevent serious illness. If you catch cold or cut yourself and develop an infection, you may not have the strength to fight it off.

Remember the stories your grand-mother (mother, father, great-grandparents, or someone) told you about children "in the old days" dying from pneumonia or influenza that most people today would survive quite easily? Well, back in those days, there weren't drugs to fight the diseases, so even healthy immune systems were sometimes unable to beat the germs. But your immune system isn't healthy right now, so it could happen to you today. Be careful with your body while your immune system is sup-pressed. You don't want to be cured of your cancer only to die from a cold!

Did we sound like mothers-in-law preaching to you about keeping your house clean, or raising your children our way? We repeated ourselves about a few issues. That was intentional and part of our job. If we sounded like we were carping, fine. We ARE mothers-in-law, just not yours, and we ARE telling you all this for your own good. So, pay attention and do as you are told. We can't open your mail, critique your cooking, or come for long, annoying visits, but we can be and are concerned about your health. We are not over-exaggerating or overreacting. We've "Been There, Done It".

Learn from our mistakes and those of the other patients who have so generously offered their experiences as a help to others. We ask you to think about your actions and those of the people around you and be wise about your health. *We want you to survive and live a long time!*

We have made "signs" that you can tear out, reproduce, whatever you'd like. One is for your home and the other for your place of work. The work sign is formatted for an office, but you can adapt it to fit the job situation you have. Post these signs in a visible spot and they can help to keep you healthy.

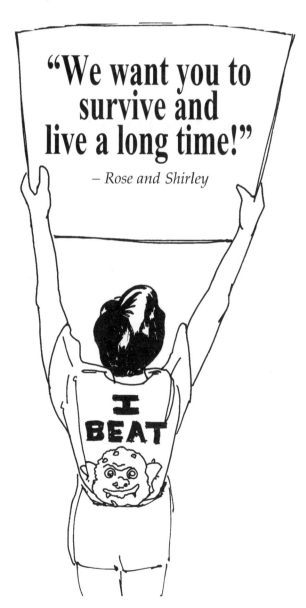

Use the following sheets as a guide. Change them to fit <u>your</u> needs.

THANKS FOR YOUR HELP

Even though I would like to, I can't shake your hand or give you a welcome hug until my immune system is stronger.

During treatment, I may need to work in a mask and gloves. I am not impersonating a doctor! My immune system is impaired.

Please don't stop by if you are sick or think you may be coming down with something.

Please do not stop by if you or your children have been recently immunized for flu or other diseases. You can pass the viruses on to me.

Please don't use my phone, pencils, pens, or other supplies from my desk when I'm not here. Germs are very dangerous for me right now.

Don't be afraid to stop by if you're healthy and say hello! I am doing great and would like to chat with you.

For the Home

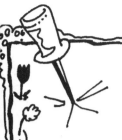

Daily Do's

I will disinfect every germ that even comes remotely close to me.

I will avoid contact with sickness.

I will stay out of crowds... even if there is a big sale at the mall!

I will eat well, drink lots of pure water and get plenty of rest.

I will take control of my day, my illness and my life.

I will love myself and not be angry about my illness and what is happening in my life.

I will find beauty in the day and savor it.

I will laugh every chance I get.

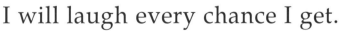

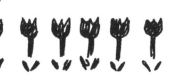

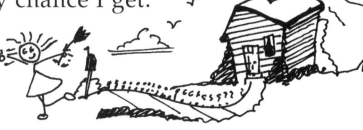

Helping Hands

Taking care of a loved one for weeks, or even years can be emotionally and physically draining. No matter how much they love you, the strain can cause resentment. The best way for both the caregiver and you to get through the situation is to start by:

Understanding your illness and resulting condition.
Knowing what symptoms and physical changes to expect.
Knowing what effect medications will have.
Determining how much assistance you will need and for how long.

You may need assistance temporarily after surgery with meal preparation or home upkeep. Ask family and friends to help out so you don't over load any one person. You'll find most of your loved ones will gladly volunteer. The community may offer special programs for temporary or long-term assistance. Ask your discharge nurse at the hospital for information and help.

You can also explore care-giving assistance through your insurance company. The local chapter of the American Cancer Society can also direct you. Nursing services have a variety of personnel who can help with all levels of home care. They have staff that can help with ostomy care, enteral feeding, chemotherapy, or even just daily meals. They also offer staff that can help you around the house, with shopping, taking you to the doctor, or other tasks.

If you do need a lot of attention, remember both you and your caregiver are in a stressful situation. You must deal with your condition, but your helper has to deal with you and the new routine as well as their own life's demands. When you can, give them a break. A few minutes to themselves or a walk in the fresh air may be good for both of you.

Remember to look for the humor in the midst of a tough situation and appreciate everything that is done for you.

Strategy #5: Keeping a Positive Image

You are what you think. The thoughts that you have over your lifetime become the truths that you believe. "I am short, friendly and hate spiders." You can have conscious thoughts such as, "I am having a good time", or unconscious thoughts such as, "Sometimes the world seems overwhelming". Don't sabotage your recovery. Keep your mind on positive images and thoughts. Remember happy times or picture yourself on vacation; don't focus continuously on your cancer. If you keep a sunny outlook, you will radiate warmth and make friends envious of your glow.

Start each day in front of the mirror. Get up out of bed, or have the mirror next to your bed and take a look at yourself. We want you to repeat a positive, esteem-building affirmation before you take your first step out into the new day. Try the ones that we used. (Center of page).

Affirmations can work wonders if you really believe what you are saying. Give them a try, make up your own, and start each day with beautiful thoughts. This may sound silly, but if you want to look good, you have to feel good about yourself. If you say loving, positive words back to yourself in the mirror, you may just convince yourself that what you say is true.

I am so happy to be alive.
I will cherish this day.
I will not let cancer
ruin this day.
Today will be a great day.
I will get through this.
I will be well.
My family/friends love me.
God loves me,
I am in his loving care.
I have faith that He will see me
through this.

I used to do this every day, even before I got sick. I said things like, "Okay, Rose, you look really great this morning. I do like your hair stuck to the side of your head like that." Or, "You will have a great day today even if those eyes are a little puffy." Or, my favorite, "I am a good woman. I did not physically attack my husband last night when he asked me what I was doing in my spare time." It works. I left the house with a smile on my face, a husband still alive at dawn, and an exciting day ahead of me. — Rose

---

Look good, feel good. We all feel better when we look good, and this is especially true for cancer patients. We've got some ideas for you to help you look good and feel better.

Beauty is skin deep, as the saying goes, so this is your opportunity to put those words to work. Perhaps some of your natural beauty is laying low and you need to wake it up. Although your outward appearance is really of little importance, it tends to be a big issue for many women.

Work hard to maintain your inner beauty and outwardly you will look wonderful. However, we know how it feels to have your personal "look" compromised, so here are a few ideas that may help.

Skin

Surgery and treatments can turn your skin into the Mojave Desert. Your definition of dry skin may take on a whole new meaning. Don't worry; you may just need to increase the grease. Vitamin E, aloe, pure oils, even olive oil are great for the skin, the more natural a product you can use, the better for your skin.

Remembering that your skin is your largest organ and will be absorbing whatever you put on it, keep the chemicals to a minimum. You will probably need to experiment a little to determine what is best for you. There are many drug store and cosmetic counter lotions and creams that will feel great. If you can make it to a health food store, check out their all-natural creams.

Aloe plants provide a soothing gel that can be used alone, or added to other creams. The fewer chemicals you absorb into your body while it is working hard to make you well, the better off you will be.

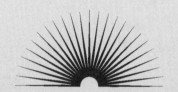

Look Good... Feel Better

One company, Look Good ... Feel Better offers a free non-medical public service program that helps women with cancer cope with the image problems created by chemotherapy side effects. If you're having self-esteem problems, this group may be of help to you. It is comprised of partners in the Cosmetic, Toiletry, and Fragrance Association, The American Cancer Society, and the National Cosmetology Association. They schedule group or one-on-one sessions to help you regain confidence you may have temporarily lost. The service is available in Canada, Australia, New Zealand, United Kingdom, and the U.S.

Look Good... Feel Better can be reached through their toll free number, **800-395-LOOK** or call your local American Cancer Society office.

I mixed vitamin E capsules with my health food store creams. It was a little heavy, but kept my skin soft. Remember to wash your face with warm or cool water. Water is wonderful for your skin. Splash cool water on your face during the day. It is very refreshing. Just pat your skin dry gently and never rub or scrub. Treat yourself with care. — Rose.

Hair

Hair loss is the process in which you spend a given number of minutes or days watching your lovely hair fill your comb, fall on the floor, lay on your pillow and stick to your clothing. The crying period over lost locks can span minutes or days. If you are on a treatment that will cause your hair to fall out, *be prepared*. There is no easy way around this issue; you're not going to like being bald. Hair loss is extremely difficult to adjust to psychologically and emotionally. Some treatments cause "fall out" in only a few days, others take weeks.

You may be on a treatment plan that causes *all* of your hair to leave you, or only some of it.

Fortunately, not everyone suffers alopecia (hair loss). Your doctor will be able to tell you if your treatment will have this side effect. Believe it or not, doctors can also tell you when it will happen — almost to the day! Waiting and watching is nearly as difficult to endure as the actual hair loss. But as hard as it may be for you to believe this, the shock factor does fade once the hair loss actually happens.

I sat up one morning in the hospital to find that a large portion of my hair had stayed behind on my pillow. Even though the nurses had forewarned me this would happen, it did not help. I thought I was prepared, but I just did not realize how "attached" to my hair I was, and so I began to cry. Two of the nurses came to console me and helped me fashion a scarf to wear over my semi-bald head. I had too much hair left to wear my wig comfortably, but not enough to look presentable. By the next morning, the remaining hair was gone. Time for the wig. However, the wig was not very practical for me, since I was bedridden so much of the time and while I slept, it would relocate on my head into strange positions. So I relied on my autographed baseball hat to keep my head warm and make myself more presentable to visitors. The rest of the time, I simply went au natural. — Shirley

---

Try to keep your finger off the panic button. If your hair does fall out, you have options. You may choose to flaunt your dome. Try interesting earrings and a variety of hats and scarves.

A company called: **Look of Love, International** offers many unique and wonderful options, as noted in the illustrations on this page. You can contact this New Jersey Company at **(908) 572-3033.**

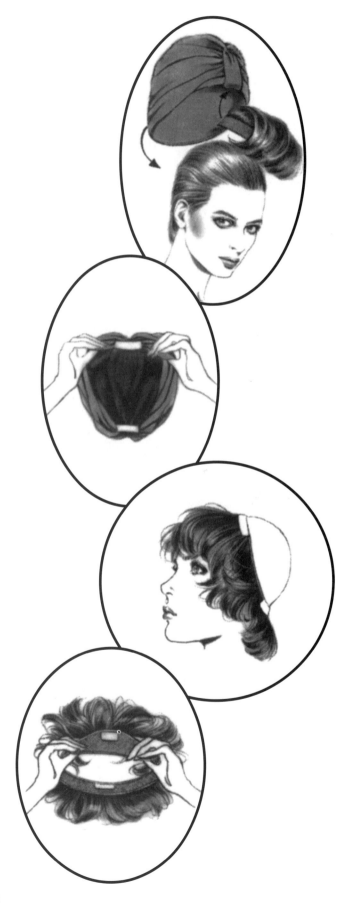

Another great company, that offers alternatives, is **Hats with Heart, Inc.**

They offer a selection of beautiful hats for women, as well as attractive, natural looking bangs, which attach to any of their headgear. The look is fabulous! Call or write for a brochure. They are located at 10271 South 1300 East, Suite 166, Sandy, Utah 84094. For the nearest retailer that carries these products, or to order a catalog, contact Hats with Heart at **1 - (800) 708-0066.**

Look at this as a fashion challenge. We've all had bad hair days and made it work somehow. This is obviously the ultimate bad hair day, but you can handle it.

I have lost my hair twice. Neither time was I brave or OK with it. I did not comb or move it around any more than I had to during the loss period. I figured 'one more day with hair', even if it was a tussled mess. After a week of denial and the 'no-touch' policy, I actually got sick and tired of cleaning up the mess it left behind. So, when I was sure it was all going to go, I just brushed out the stragglers. Once it was out, I just got used to it and went on with getting well. After all, it was going to grow back! A little advice: If you have long hair, cut it short before it begins to fall out. It won't seem so monumental a loss. It's a psychological ploy, but it works. I decided to look on the lighter side of this baldness thing. When friends asked about my hair or wanted to see my head, I offered to let them autograph it. They usually declined because they thought I was kidding. I was not. Just think how nice a fully signed head would be. It would be as though you had a get well card to look at every trip to the mirror. —Rose

---

Another great look is the ever-faithful baseball cap, which can be purchased in any one of a trillion colors, logos, and materials. Support your favorite team or cover the hat in patches, pins, or whatever. You can purchase plain (no emblem) baseball-style hats also.

Use your imagination and create your own unique statement; however, try to avoid the fisherman's look — fishhooks in your hat are not such a good idea under the circumstances.

"Explore everything around you, penetrate to the furthest limits of human knowledge, and always you will come up with something inexplicable in the end. It is called life."

- Albert Schweitzer

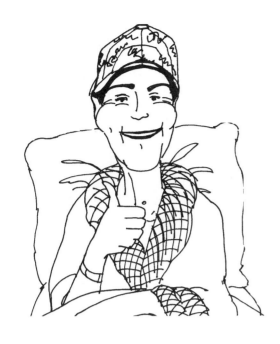

As I mentioned earlier, I spent a lot of time in my hospital bed, which made it difficult to for me keep on a scarf or a wig; when I slept, they would get turned around or fall off! So I slept au natural (my head, that is) and kept a plain white baseball-style hat on the top of the bed for handy access should a guest arrive. By the time the visitor had knocked, donned his/her requisite mask and entered my room, the hat was sitting on my head, making all present feel more comfortable. As an added touch, I asked everyone to autograph the hat for me. No one ever refused my request, and I'm very proud of all the signatures on that hat! — Shirley

Wigs seem to be the most popular antidote to hair loss. In most cities you can locate a wig shop that caters to cancer patients. If you are unsure, ask the home health department at the hospital or the American Cancer Society and they will provide the referrals. Wig companies advertise in the back of ladies' magazines and you can order from a catalog if all else fails. There are many wig styles available. Although some women prefer a wig that makes them look exactly like they did before their hair loss, no one is pigeonholed into their old look. For some of us, looking exactly the same is important. For others, not. If you do decide to purchase a wig ahead of time, save a clump of hair from the "big fall out" and take it with you. You can match the wig to your natural hair color.

You might want to experiment at the wig shop before your hair leaves the premises. Take someone with you to give you a second opinion, or bring along a picture of yourself to help the personnel at the wig shop match your look. We strongly suggest that you bring along a friend. Have fun trying on different styles. Don't limit yourself to wigs that reflect your current look. It is a great opportunity to change your hair color or style.

My first time hairless, I tried a totally different look. I went Big Hair Curly Blonde. It was fun. Most people never guessed it was a wig. In fact, I found the look was very appealing to workers at construction sites. It was "hoot-and-howl" soliciting. For my second adventure into the world of the hairless, I tried the old, curly look. Ouch! Really awful. Then I found THE wig. Just call me "straight bob Rose", the little sophisticate. It is good to change your look sometimes. — Rose

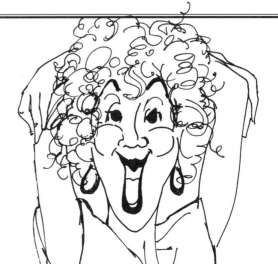

I did not plan ahead for my hair loss, nor did I feel adventurous, so I ended up looking a bit frumpy with a very unflattering wig. However, I rectified the problem after I finally got out of the hospital by splurging on another wig. It looked just like my regular hairstyle, which was what I wanted. I needed to look as much like "my old self" as possible. However, my one-year-old granddaughter had seen me bald, so she knew that it was a wig and she loved to pull it off and rub my head with her soft little hands. I did not mind a bit, but other people were not always as thrilled when she tried to pull their hair off! It took her a while to understand that only Grandma had removable hair! — Shirley

Wig shops can trim the wig to fit your features or you can take it to your hair stylist and have she or he create your new look. Try wearing it a few times before you lose your hair. You will feel more comfortable with it when the hair loss occurs. It will help you get used to it.

In fact, even though the doctor called the Fall Out just about to the day, I still worried that my hair would just drop to my feet some day at work, so I started wearing my wig about a week early. When my hair finally went, I was already used to wearing the wig. — Rose

Friends will get used to you with the wig and after a short while won't even notice it anymore. If your budget will allow, you should have two wigs for convenience. (Medical insurance policies usually cover the cost of one wig only). Unless you think you will feel like washing, setting and styling, or dropping your wig off at the hairdresser, look for synthetic hair. A human hair wig can cost as much as $500. A nice synthetic wig, pre-styled, can be less than $100. You can wash your wigs in wig shampoo. Don't use regular shampoo or any other cleaner. The wig shampoo keeps the shine, color and style looking new. Other cleaners strip the shine off and the wigs become flyaway. Most wigs dry within just a few hours of washing. Be sure to follow directions for care. The wig will last longer. One benefit to a wig: you can get ready to go out in half the time. Shine your head with creams or oils, and pop on the wig. A couple of fluffs and you are out the door.

Your hair may not fall out, but it could be damaged by treatments. Avoid abusing it with over-brushing, hair sprays, dyes, permanents, mousse, blow-dryers and curling irons. Take it easy whenever possible. It is also nice to sleep on a silky pillowcase. The case will cut down on breakage.

Shampoos that are designed to remove perspiration, soap and other buildups in hair follicles are great for keeping the scalp in good condition. Health food stores, department store make-up counters, and your local pharmacies will provide you with a good selection of products.

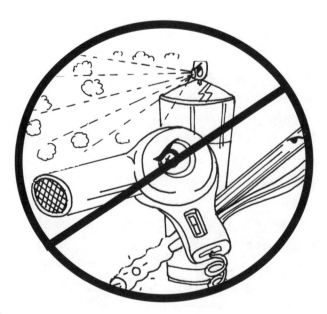

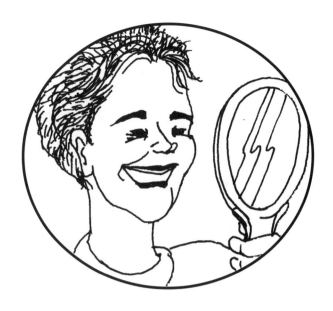

Hair Regrowth:
A process in which
you watch with great joy
as your hair returns.

Often, your regrowth hair will be slightly different than the hair you lost. Many people experience natural curls for the first time — although this is usually a temporary change. Your new hair will be very soft at first, and may even be a different shade of your previous color. You may find that during the first inch or two of regrowth your wig will become increasingly uncomfortable to wear, especially if you live in a warm climate. Try to go wig-free as much as possible — around the house, on weekends, etc. You may want to get your hair trimmed as it grows back, to begin forming your new hairstyle.

As my hair grew back, it did not all return at the same rate, so I started to develop a "shag-rug" look that was less-than-attractive. My hairstylist kept it trimmed so that I maintained a semblance of style during regrowth. At her own insistence, Fran came to my house for the first trim; and the for the next, she opened her salon early so that she could cut my hair before anyone else came in. She was protecting me from any embarrassment I might have felt at being seen in public with my lush half inch of hair, and from the germ-count of a salon full of customers. Not everyone is lucky enough to have such a considerate hairstylist, but I'll bet if you ask yours, he or she will be very accommodating. — Shirley

Face

On to the face... cancer treatments and surgery can make you look pasty. Get ahead of the problem. Get down to basics with your skin. Wash with gentle products and pat your skin dry. If you feel your skin is holding up pretty well, exfoliate to remove dead skin and treat yourself to a facial at a salon or in the privacy of your own bathroom. Oatmeal is an all-natural and inexpensive facial scrub that works great. Try cucumbers on the eyelids to calm puffiness. Olive oil works great at softening the skin. If your eyes are puffy, use Preparation H on them; it is an old trick of professional make-up artists. It smells funny, but it really works. Just use a little dab under the eye. Buy foundation that is a shade more colorful than your regular look, with perhaps a lighter color for under your eyes. Try mixing and matching. Use a little blush for that natural, rosy-cheeked look. Adjust your color palette to suit your mood and clothing. Look good and it may help you feel good!

We recommend for women who really want a pick-me-up; go to a department store make-up counter and have one of the consultants suggest a program. If you don't want to spend a fortune, choose the items you positively must have and then buy the generic brands from your regular sources. Keep your make-up kit handy and begin the paint job. If the eyebrows go, find a soft pencil and draw them back in. False eyelashes work great if you have a little coordination and perseverance. If your nails chip or become softer, have a manicure or try false nails. Maintenance is so important. If you can keep your appearances up to your normal standards, neither you nor anyone else will notice the changes in you. The closer you look to your old self, the better you will feel.

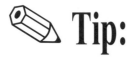

Tip:

Discard mascara after a month. It may contain animal fats, which can develop bacterial growth. Read ingredients on all make-up for your protection. If you are normally prone to eye infections, you may want to discontinue eye make-up during treatment.

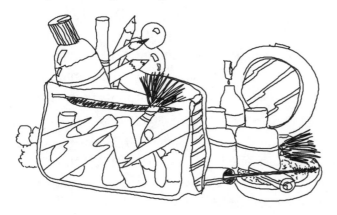

After you have that "I've just had my face blow-torched look" that comes from the chemo-induced hair loss, look at a picture of yourself (perhaps you should take a close-up shot before you start treatments). You can use the picture to build those tricky eyebrows back into their natural arch. I missed the mark the first

couple of times and looked like Ming the Merciless of Flash Gordon fame! I think the funniest part of facial hair loss is the nose hair that goes too. Now that is one weird thing to look at. Your nostril openings look like two black holes in space. You can really see quite far up there! — Rose

Body

Now to the body... you may see some changes. Perhaps surgery or treatment changed your appearance. So what? You are still the same person. You have morphed to a new and improved you. If you have surgery scars or have lost some part of your body, try thinking of yourself as now being more highly evolved. You can now function with fewer parts. How many times have you admired someone's appearance and not even noticed facial or body flaws, scars, speech problems, or physical limitations? That happens because you see the beauty in the whole person, not in the individual aspects of their persona. Turn that theory around and use it on yourself.

After my mastectomy I used to tell people I had a more difficult time keeping abreast of a situation. Oh, and it was not so easy to get you-know-what caught in a wringer. When I had two tummy cuts, I decided to use them as conversation pieces. You know , like you could connect the lines on my torso and find the map to the lost continent of Atlantis. — Rose

The point is — don't focus on negatives. Turn them around and see the sunny side of life. You will feel a lot better if you do. Each day is a gift from God.

Remember: He loves you and you have Shirley and Rose pulling for you too.

You are the same loving, wonderful person you were before cancer.

Remember that.

It is possible you could be dealing with your cancer as a chronic problem for many years. Get used to the changes it may bring with it. They are really very small when you consider your "big picture". We'll bet that most of your friends and family won't even notice the difference in you at all. With all that we have been through, we are still the same as we always were.

Friends still think of us in the same way — crazy and short. No one even noticed our new, streamlined bodies! **Love yourself. You deserve it.**

All right... our guess is that you have gotten just a little lazy since all this cancer stuff has started. Understandable, but don't make a habit of it. You will feel and look better if you try a little exercise. Go for a walk. It really helps.

After my ovarian surgery, I could only walk two houses down the street and then had to drag myself back home. I sure felt better, though, taking those few steps. The fresh air was great, I got the blood flowing, and I felt like I was walking back in the direction of normal life. — Rose

While I was in the hospital undergoing my leukemia treatment, it was a major project for me to go for a walk. Everywhere I went, my handy IV infusion pump named George (it needed a name, since it was my constant companion) had to go with me. At the lowest point during my treatment, just getting out of bed was a major accomplishment, and

lugging George around took a lot of effort. But as my strength returned, my husband was very persistent that I go for a walk at least once a day; preferably three times. I think we may have set some kind of mileage record as we walked endlessly around the nurses' station every day; me, with my baseball hat, mask, and five-wheeled pal George, and my husband Russ acting as my coach and cheerleader. The only thing missing, besides any semblance of speed, was fresh air; and as soon as I got home, I went outside just to walk up and down the driveway and smell the fresh air. (It was about 10^0 F outside, so I did not dare go for a "real" walk, but wow did that cold fresh air smell wonderful!!) — Shirley

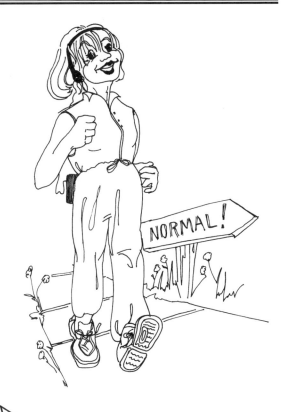

Tip: If you are going to have a professional manicure, bring your own emery boards, orange sticks and clippers. Do not trim your cuticles. The salon may be a source of germs. If you want to give yourself a manicure, keep your equipment clean and disinfected.

Clothing

The best-dressed cancer patients are those who actually decide to get out of their pajamas and put on some real clothes. There is no argument from us that it is really comfy and consoling to lay around in your robe or loose, baggy clothing. That does feel great. Even putting on make-up or daily bathing can become a "not every day" thing. If you need to do that for a while, do so. On the other hand, regaining some normalcy in your day-to-day life will make you feel better. Perhaps try a nicer outfit or suit once in a while and go out for lunch. If you can't go out, invite someone in. Make it easy on yourself: invite them over and ask them to bring themselves *and* the food. Sometimes, just cleaning up and looking like your old self can do wonders for the spirit. You may notice that the cancer really hasn't changed you at all. You are still the good-looking devilette you always were!

Breast surgery can seem disfiguring, but the amount of cellulite packed onto my thighs is much uglier than my reconfigured breast set-up. (Just a personal note from Rose!) If you have lost a breast, there are many options. Please do not think you will never wear a sweater again. You can choose from both breast reconstruction and breast forms that slip into your bra.

This is very important: don't jump at the first suggestion made by your doctor. He may be more comfortable with a certain procedure that he uses on most of his breast cancer patients (cookie-cutter medical procedures). There are several types of reconstruction done, including surgical implants and flap reconstruction.

The surgical implant method uses a

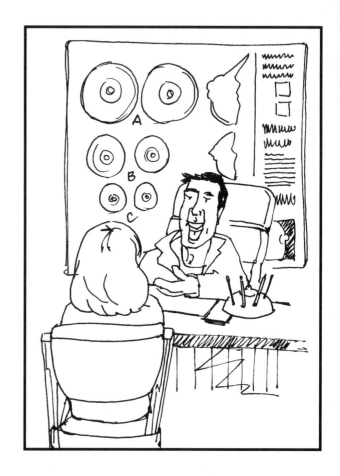

saline or silicone implant similar to the type used for cosmetic surgery (a.k.a. boob jobs). You may start the procedure immediately after the mastectomy in the operating room. Your plastic surgeon will place a tissue expander under the muscle. The tissue expander is used to stretch the muscle and surrounding tissue to accommodate the implant. Surgeons can create a very realistic breast with this method. The tissue expander is taken out, probably after your immune system is back in order again, and replaced with the implant. This means more surgery. If you want nipple reconstruction, the surgeon may take a strip of skin from the area where your thigh meets your torso. With plastic surgery magic, they turn that into the most realistic nipple you have ever seen. However, that is another surgery. The reconstruction is not totally painless, but mostly "uncomfortable" describes it.

Flap reconstruction is a little more complicated. The plastic surgeon has to relocate muscle, fat, and skin which is taken from an alternate site on the body. He may go hunting on the tummy, back or buttocks. Surgeons are able to tunnel fat from the abdomen and place it in the breast area. This method is sometimes preferred because the finished product is all you, inside and out. You would still have to have the nipple surgery, too. The important thing to remember is that you can have reconstruction done any time you want, even years after the mastectomy. Your doctor may recommend that you wait. Generally, it is up to you. Just remember that you need a plastic surgeon. *Don't let anyone tell you otherwise.* Visit several and learn the current innovations for breast reconstruction and you may find a procedure suited to you. You can always wear an external prosthesis for a while to see how you like it. Ask questions. Make a decision based on knowledge and preference. Hats with Heart, Inc. (listed on page 102 and on the resource page at the end of this chapter) also offers a specialty lingerie catalog of post-mastectomy solutions. The catalog is entitled "Feminine Image".

Clothing may have to change some, but usually only minor adjustments are required. If you've had surgery, you may temporarily need to avoid clothing that is restrictive or irritating in the area of the surgery. Or you may need to wear loose - fitting clothes that you can put on without physical difficulty. Ostomy patients usually believe that they will have to wear different clothing, but this is rarely true. Many ostomy pouches made today are not bulky and do not show under even the most stylish or form-fitting clothing. Try to keep your weight down, for obvious reasons, and also because it makes the appliance fit more properly. Some women find cotton knit or stretch underpants give them the support and security they desire. If you have a catheter in your chest or abdomen, wear soft comfortable clothing. Luckily, that is the style. You will look so chic.

The weight gain, which usually accompanies the return of a healthy appetite following surgery, has more effect on clothing choice than anything else.

Try adding a little color to your wardrobe. It is cheery and will brighten up your look. Stand up straight! (Words from childhood?). Do it. Your clothes will look better and you will actually feel better. Cancer likes to make you look weak and tired. It will try to make you walk the walk and talk the talk of a sick person. I think it is part of the evil tricks it plays on you. Don't stand bent over. Stand up to the challenge. Think of how you looked before your illness. Assume the stature of a survivor. Put your shoulders back, take a few deep breaths and put a smile on your face. You can get through this without it breaking your spirit.

my own resources

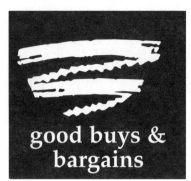

good buys & bargains

(This is your chance to help others. If you find any good resources, e-mail or fax us at 407/330-3433, and we will share your finds.)
KEEP THIS HANDY FOR YOUR USE.

_____
MANUFACTURER'S NAME

_____
MAILING ADDRESS

_____
CITY   STATE   ZIP CODE

_____
PRODUCT DESCRIPTION

_____
MANUFACTURER/DISTRIBUTOR TELEPHONE NO.

_____
MANUFACTURER'S NAME

_____
MAILING ADDRESS

_____
CITY   STATE   ZIP CODE

_____
PRODUCT DESCRIPTION

_____
MANUFACTURER/DISTRIBUTOR TELEPHONE NO.

_____
MANUFACTURER'S NAME

_____
MAILING ADDRESS

_____
CITY   STATE   ZIP CODE

_____
PRODUCT DESCRIPTION

_____
MANUFACTURER/DISTRIBUTOR TELEPHONE NO.

Self-Image Resource Sheet

Hair

Look of Love International
1913 Route 27, Edison, NJ 08817
(908) 572-3033

Hats with Heart, Inc.
10271 South 1300 East, Suite 166,
Sandy, Utah 84094.
For the nearest retailer that carries these products, or to order a catalog, call 1 - (800) 708-0066.

Other

Alra Oncology Care
Non-metallic, gentle, non-irritating stearate based stick deodorant which contains natural antibacterial ingredients, no petroleum derived ingredients, no alcohol, or metallic salts.
1-800-832-8311

'Feminine Image', Hats with Heart, Inc.
10271 South 1300 East, Suite 166
Sandy, Utah 84094
1-800-708-0066

Look Good... Feel Better

A program developed by the Cosmetic, Toiletry and Fragrance Association, the National Cosmetology Association and the American Cancer Society - designed to help patients take care of their hair, skin, nails, and appearance.
1-800-395-LOOK

NEUE Medical Products
711 South Main Street,
Burbank, CA 91506
Offers ALRA Oncology Care Products and NEUE Antibacterial Products, including lotions, shampoo, aloe vera gel, etc.
(818) 563-4869 or (800) 832-8311

Strategy #6: Maintaining Control of Your Mind & Body Through Nutrition & Exercise

We first thought a separate chapter on exercise and one on nutrition would be the most effective. The more we researched, the clearer it became to us that they go hand in hand.

Nutrition

After decades of research, scientists and doctors have come to the conclusion that up to 50 percent of all cancers may be linked to diet. So what you eat and don't eat can tilt the odds of escaping certain types of cancer in your favor. Over one hundred food compounds have been credited with the ability to fight cancer. These are some of the best cancer-fighting foods:

All cruciferous vegetables, including broccoli, Brussels sprouts, cabbage, cauliflower, rutabagas, turnips

All dark green and yellow fruits and vegetables, especially apricots, carrots, pumpkin, spinach, sweet potatoes

All whole grains

Beans (dried)

Bran (wheat)

Citrus fruits (grapefruit, oranges, tangerines)

Fish, especially mackerel, salmon, tuna

Melons (cantaloupe)

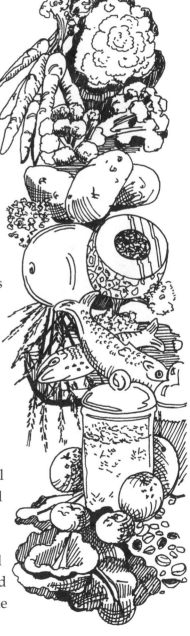

Milk (low fat)

Nuts

Onions

Papayas

Potatoes

Rice (brown)

Salad greens

Tropical fruits (guavas)

The National Cancer Institute has issued dietary guidelines for cancer prevention, which include cruciferous vegetables and low fat foods. What you eat may be what you are.

A nutritious diet is vital for keeping your body working at its best. During treatment good nutrition is even more important. If you eat well during treatment you will probably cope with the side effects of the drugs better. A healthy diet will keep up your strength and help rebuild tissue that the treatments may harm.

Now that you have some background on the nutrition subject, we might as well start with the topic we all hate to talk about: our weight. Treatments will do one of three things to your weight!

1. Nothing
2. Thin you down
3. Fatten you up
(oh yes, it happens all the time)

If you tolerate your treatments well, you may not notice a weight change. It is possible that between the cancer, surgery and treatment you may drop some weight. It is not permanent and will return to normal as you get better. If you lose too much weight and need to put it back on, check with the nutrition professional on your team, or go to the health food store and ask for their recommendations. Be sure to clear with your doctors any unusual drinks or pills that are suggested to you. We don't necessarily recommend the dietitian at the hospital. They tend to recommend white bread, butter and milk shakes. A balanced diet, designed to work within your bodies current needs and capabilities, is what you need. You may even get lucky enough to have milk shakes written into your plan. If your nutritional guidance is currently limited to the dietitian at the hospital, go into your community and search for someone trained in supporting cancer patients during and after treatment. You may be forced to go out

of your area. Check health food stores; some may have nutritionists on staff or know someone in your area that can help. The Internet is loaded with information on healthy eating for cancer patients. If you can not find or afford a nutrition specialist work with the American Cancer Society, your hospital, and the information you gather from them to develop a healthy meal plan for you during treatment. There are many resources to check with. Whatever you do, definitely get a strong nutrition plan together.

Be sure to clear with your doctors any unusual drinks, foods or pills that are suggested to you.

After my hysterectomy, cancer debulking, and colon resection, the only foods I could eat were soft and bland. For three months the nutritionist suggested that all I eat was mashed potatoes, white bread, mayonnaise, whipped cream, and turkey slices. (Well, maybe not just those few items, but pretty close.) I had a touchy tummy and could not digest fruits and vegetables. This is harsh news to a vegetarian. I was getting desperate enough to sell off family heirlooms for a piece of fresh produce.

Finally, I gave up and ate some vegetables. Yummie! They disagreed with my digestion for the next three months, but oh, what flavor in a fresh tomato! I had to experiment to find foods I could tolerate. If you do have a special diet, stick to it, but start with good, healthy foods and go easy on the snacks and desserts. — Rose

Surprisingly, your weight may go up during treatment. Today's anti-nausea medications for chemo and radiation treatments have stopped many of the nausea problems usually associated with cancer treatment. The new medications available keep the "pukies" down to nothing.

However, you may feel sluggish or flu-like some days. It is really easy to lay around and graze in the fridge. Hence, we have weight gain. Don't be too hard on yourself. It feels good to eat a little too much. Just don't get carried away. Remember that sweets can cause metabolic problems and caffeine and sodas wash away vitamins. You can get the normalcy back into your weight when you feel better. Your body may need a little fat to keep the furnace stoked during this time of great stress. A little extra now might not hurt. Eat sensibly and limit the fatty snacks. Remember it's easier to put on the weight than take it off.

Your immune system, (cells and proteins that fight foreign invaders like virus, bacteria and cancer), is working hard each day to kill off cells that do not belong in your body. Immune cells come from your bone marrow. Your marrow incubates and gives birth to millions of little red and white blood cells. The red cells carry oxygen, but the white cells are the basis of your immune system. The white cells are your own personal army that attacks foreign invaders like viruses, bacteria and cancer. White blood cells called macrophage (meaning "eater") gobble up the enemy invaders. These natural killer cells constantly guard against cells that have gone bad, such as

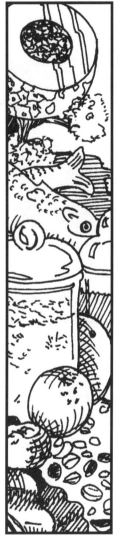

tumor cells. Tumors are cells that have gone out of control and need to be stopped. When the macrophage have done their job, they let the other white cells, lymphocytes, out. They are your Special Forces Team. They can be either T-cells or B-cells. B-cells stay in the bone marrow, evolve into plasma cells and discharge antibodies to fight disease and infection. The T-cells directly attack the enemy cells. Somehow the lymphocytes can identify a traitor in their ranks and they go in for the kill.

When your immune system is not working well, you will most likely be ill. It is important to maintain the highest level of immune function during treatment. Your body is waging a terrible war inside trying to defeat the cancer. You are the reinforcements it is waiting for. Don't let it down. You have to help by providing your body with the weapons it needs to win the war.

Basic nutrition guidelines suggest a certain amount of fat, calories, vitamins and minerals. The amount in each category swings from an average as established by the USDA to heavier doses of particular nutrients prescribed to combat deficiencies.

The National Cancer Institute recommends the consumption of at least five fruits and vegetables a day in a program called "5 a Day for Better Health". Your local supermarket will probably have informative pamphlets on the program and suggestions on how to get your 5 a Day. The USDA created "The Food Guide Pyramid" to support consuming a range of foods from the major food groups to provide your body with the right amount of nutrients and calories. The supermarket will have information for you on the Pyramid.

You may not know of the resources at your disposal at the supermarket. Most of the bigger supermarkets have nutritionists affiliated with them or on staff. They can provide you with good nutrition information from many sources. If your treatment causes diarrhea, you may need to cut back on high-fiber foods such as vegetables, fruits, cereals, and whole grains for a while.

During treatment you may need special dietary supplementation. Your immune system is under constant attack from pollution, tobacco smoke and other environmental poisons. Adding to the problem are toxic debris from undigested foods like processed foods, sugars, and harsh chemicals, which create free *radicals* that circulate in your system causing problems. These wastes travel through your bloodstream, destroy normal metabolism, may even damage your DNA, and add to the work your body goes through to keep you healthy. Wherever these waste molecules come from, you want to get rid of them quickly. You can help your body fight the free radicals and the treatment effects with *antioxidants*. These nutrients, which boost your immune response, are found in many of the foods you should be eating. Some vitamins like A, C, E and the minerals selenium and zinc fight and destroy free radicals.

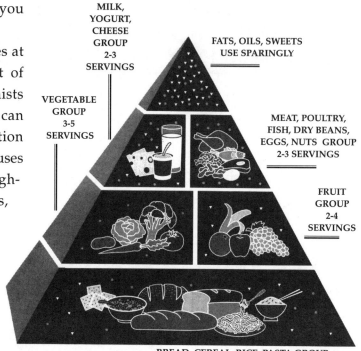

The USDA created "The Food Guide Pyramid" to support consuming a range of foods from the major food groups to provide your body with the right amount of nutrients and calories.

To order a copy of "The Food Guide Pyramid" booklet, send a $1 check or money order made out to the Superintendent of Documents to: Consumer Information Center, Department 159-Y, Pueblo, CO 81009.

U.S. dept. of Agriculture, Human Nutrition Information Service, August 1992, Leaflet No. 572

The following list will give you natural sources of these nutrients:

⚬ **Beta Carotene (soluble A)** - fish liver oils, yellow and green fruits and vegetables, carrots, tomatoes, spinach, peppers, alfalfa, asparagus, beets, dandelion greens, garlic, watercress, cherries, peaches, kale, parsley, pumpkin, yellow squash, turnip greens, mustard, papayas, spirulina, broccoli, watermelon and apricots. Dark green vegetables get an A+.

Vitamin C - Citrus fruits, strawberries, melons, leafy green vegetables, tomatoes, potatoes, asparagus, avocados, beet greens, broccoli, Brussels sprouts, cantaloupe, collards, currants, grapefruit, kale, lemons, mangos, mustard greens, onions, ranges, papayas, watercress, tomatoes, spinach, radishes, green peas, rose hips, and turnip greens.

Vitamin E - Whole grains, brown rice, wheat germ, oats, soy beans, parsley, asparagus, cold-pressed olive oil and other vegetable oils, dark green leafy vegetables, nuts and seeds, legumes. Dry beans, cornmeal, eggs, desiccated liver, milk, oatmeal, organ meats, sweet potatoes.

Selenium - Whole grain cereals, Brazil nuts, brewer's yeast, wheat germ, dairy products, liver, bran, garlic, onions, broccoli, seafood, tuna, brown rice, chicken, molasses, onions, salmon and mushrooms.

Zinc - (too much can depress the immune system) - fish, legumes, soybeans, sunflower seeds, pecans, pumpkin seeds, lamb chops, sardines, brewer's yeast, egg yolks, lima beans, mushrooms, seeds, and soy lecithin.

Surgery can reduce your immune function by up to 50%. Some reports indicate that painkillers such as morphine can lower your immune power also. If your immune function is low, so are your recuperatory powers. If you are not eating a balanced diet or not eating much at all, the immune system will not work properly. You may need to increase your caloric intake after surgery and during treatment to give your body the fuel it needs to run under stress. For example: bone marrow requires 4000 calories-a-day to rebuild itself!

If you are taking a medication or radiation, ask the doctor to provide you with information on what the treatment is doing to your liver, kidneys, vitamin and mineral levels, etc. You may want to call the manufacturer of the drugs you are taking and ask them for a complete report of all the side effects and cautions on using their drug. Most of them have 800 numbers. Also, if possible, get on the Internet. There is a great deal of information for cancer patients on the Net. You may also find a chat line on the Net with other patients who are taking or have taken the drug. Get to know what is happening on the inside of your body.

Over-consumption of vitamins, minerals or specialized supplements can cause toxicity. It is critical that before you make additions to your diet, you discuss your plan with your doctor and nutrition team members. Many doctors are trained to assist you with particular nutritional problems during treatment. If your doctor is not familiar with this facet of care, and you do not have a nutrition specialist on your team, check the phone book, health food stores or even chiropractors, some of whom work with area nutritionists.

Many vitamins, such as vitamin C, which normally have few side effects in healthy individuals, can adversely affect you during treatment. Some vitamins can actually fight the chemo. We do not recommend any particular regimen of supplements. What we do recommend is thoroughly researching what will help your body withstand the treatment you are taking.

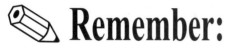

Remember:

Chemo, radiation or any drug therapy is shocking your system. If your doctor says that you don't need anything, he probably has very little nutritional education. You must take the initiative. Don't come away cured of your cancer and have problems from the damage done during treatment. And don't think these things can't happen. Survivors all have stories about the after-affects of their chemo or radiation treatments.

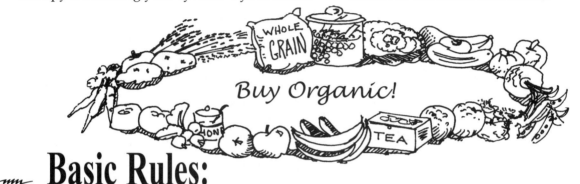

Basic Rules:

Cut down on fat, sugars, alcohol, and caffeine.

Omit salt-cured, smoked and nitrate-treated meats and processed foods.

Eat lots of whole grains, fresh fruits and vegetables.*

Try to maintain a healthy weight.

Check with your doctor. During or after certain treatments, patients must avoid fresh foods until their immune systems can tolerate the bacteria present on fresh produce.

More Basic Rules:

When shopping for foods, look for natural, fresh and organic. You want to run the cleanest fuel through your body.

Try to eat foods in their natural state when possible, if digestion and immune system will allow.

Look for naturally raised meats without antibiotics, growth hormones and other chemicals, which are added to most meat products.

Use sesame seed and cold pressed extra virgin olive oil in cooking. They have the highest smoke point before dangerous carcinogens begin forming.

Drink distilled or purified spring water when possible.

Try herbal teas; stay away from coffee and regular tea.

Cook in stainless steel cookware.

Use butter instead of margarine.

Use fresh herbs and sprouts often.

Go easy on salts.

Use apple cider vinegar instead of wine or balsamic.

~ Don'ts:

⊘ Eat process foods such as sugar, white bread, frozen meals, and chips.

⊘ Eat foods with dyes, preservatives, or artificial colors.

⊘ Drink carbonated beverages.

⊘ Eat fried foods, white rice.

⊘ Eat chocolate (Oh get real, you're gonna' cheat on this one!)

⊘ Eat canned fruits, vegetables and meats.

⊘ Eat foods too hot, cold or spicy. They may upset your system.

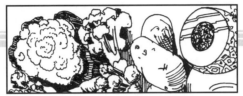

Lettuce get a New Leaf on Life!

The old adage of "You are what you eat" is really true. If you put good fuel into your car, the engine will work more efficiently and the parts will last longer. How do you put good fuel into your engine? You can cut back on saturated fats and processed foods. Organic foods offer excellent nutritional content and little or no pesticides. They cost a little more, but with a little hunting around, you can locate organic produce and prepared foods that will improve your nutritional intake. Organic foods are raised with limited amounts of pesticides and fertilizers. To be "Certified Organic" a third party has to evaluate the farmers' growing practices. California, and several other states, have strict rules for organic farming. There is a trend in the food industry to provide a wider selection of organic foods for consumers in the grocery store. If you look closely, your supermarket may have a great selection of produce, pastas, cereals, cookies (yum yum), pizzas and many other foods.

Oh yes, don't look past the tofu or soy products either when planning a healthy diet. They offer alternative protein sources. Tofu pepperoni is delicious!

If your selection of organics is limited also look for "Natural" foods. A word of caution: the federal and state governments have no official certification or regulation of the "Natural" category of foods. Currently a manufacturer can label a product "Natural" strictly for marketing purposes. One exception is the USDA, which does have a "Natural" classification for meat that adheres to their guidelines of being "minimally processed and free of artificial ingredients". Look for foods and companies that use products like whole wheat and honey or concentrated fruit juices instead of refined sugars and enriched bleached flours.

Make a concerted effort to stay away from foods that are laced with preservatives such as BHA, BHT, MSG, artificial colorings, sodium nitrates (in almost all cold cuts), saccharin and aspartame.

It sounds like a lot, but it really is easy to convert to healthy eating. There are many books available on healing foods. Pick one up at the library and give yourself and the new foods a chance.

Exercise

Even moderate exercise seems to have a cumulative effect on the immune system. To help metabolize your food, you need to stimulate your system through exercise. Don't shut the book here because you don't feel like exercising. It can come in some very easy forms that even you in your present "I don't want to" mood can handle. Some of them can be done right in your comfy chair.

Exercises can be mental and physical. What a powerful body energizer when you combine them both! Mental exercises are very simply explained, but some may take a little concentrating to accomplish. The mind is a powerful factor in your overall health. Study upon study has been done showing the relationship between the body and the mind. You have only to pick up a magazine at any given time and see articles on survivors who have cured themselves spontaneously, much to the confusion of their doctors. Positive attitude can actually raise your immune function.

The immune system is controlled by the brain, either indirectly through hormones in the blood stream, or directly through nerves and neurochemicals.

One of the most widely accepted explanations of cancer, the "surveillance" theory, states that cancer cells are developing in our bodies all the times but are normally destroyed by white blood cells before they can develop into dangerous tumors. Cancer appears when the immune system becomes suppressed and can no longer deal with this routine threat. It follows that whatever upsets the brain's control of the immune system will foster malignancy.

"Anatomical evidence for direct control of the immune system by the brain has been confirmed in studies of animals. Two groups of scientist have independently used Pavlovian conditioning techniques to change the immune response. At the University of Rochester Medical Center, psychiatrist Robert Ader and immunologist Nicholas Cohen repeatedly gave rats saccharin-sweetened water along with an immune-suppressant drug. Later they were able to 'trick' the animals into suppressing their own immune responses by giving them the sweetened water alone." – from Dr. Bernie S. Siegel's, "Love, Medicine and Miracles"

Read that again in case you did not get the full meaning. This is powerful news. You have just been given one of the keys to survival. The power may be within you.

The three types of immune boosting mental exercises we think work the best are:

1. Positive Thinking

2. Meditation

3. Guided Imagery (Visualization)

Positive thinking really sounds good, doesn't it? "I will be well again." Good thinking, but hard to convince yourself. You are probably having the same thoughts we had. "Will I be here next year?" "Will I see my family grow up?"

"Will I live or die?" There are a thousand frightening questions that will run through your mind. Let them in one side and shoo them out the other. You will not be able to stop them from coming; however, you can handle them so that they lose some of their bite. No one knows if she will be here tomorrow, let alone next year. So, focus on the positive. Your body cannot tell the difference between reality and thoughts.

Our minds automatically imagine the worst scenarios when told we have cancer. Our bodies respond to our mind's fantasies of good and bad and to actual circumstances. Cancer can make you feel helpless and chronic feelings like that can upset the body's balance. This stress is dangerous for you right now.

A study conducted at Ohio State Medical School by Dr. Janice Kiecolt-Glaser and Dr. Ronald Glaser, her husband, found that students under stress of exams showed decreased lymphocytes, which if you remember, are the white blood cell soldiers helping to destroy tumor cells. You have good doctors, you want to live really badly, and you are treating your cancer the very best way you can. Your head has to be screwed on straight and pushing forward. This relates back to Chapter One when we told you to get all negative thinkers away from you. You have to see yourself well

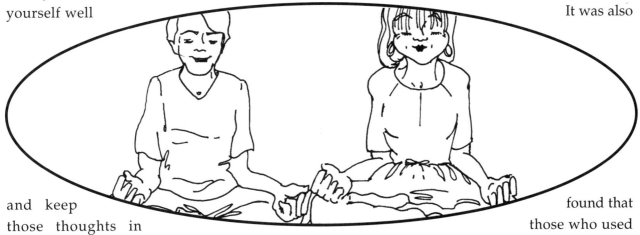

and keep those thoughts in the forefront of your mind. When the dark thoughts try to creep in, crush them with, "No I will not think of that. I will continue to do my best to get well and appreciate

every minute of every day I have on this earth."

Of the 54 heart surgery patients included in a study done at Carnegie-Mellon University, the optimists healed faster, left the hospital sooner, had less complications and heart attack reoccurrences.

A good attitude gets you farther in life and makes you feel much better about yourself.

Meditation induces a state of relaxation, although its goal is to increase awareness. It comes in many forms with names like Kundalini, Tantra, Zen and Transcendental. For our purposes, we feel that Transcendental is the easiest to begin with because it does not involve having a particular religious philosophy, outside stimulus or physical manipulation.

It can be more relaxing physiologically and psychologically than sleep. Meditation allows you to listen to the inner you and make better choices in day to day decisions, even more so now when every decision is important.

A study conducted at Harvard University found a notable drop in the frequency of headaches, colds and insomnia among regular meditators. It was also found that those who used mediation reported more positive mood states.

Meditation demands that you focus your concentration on a given task for a period of time. Your goal is to quiet your mind and to let thoughts and images run through your mind without focusing on any one of them in particular. You will have to practice.

Learning mediation techniques under your current stress levels will take a little work in the beginning; however it will make a big difference in your state of being. Your worries, health problems and everyday thoughts will fight you at first. Your mind jumps from one thought to another. It is actual work to get it to be still. With practice it will get easier. Do not get discouraged. Even the long time meditators have wandering minds.

As you get into the swing of meditating regularly, you will begin to experience physical relaxation. It is truly peaceful, and you will be encouraged by those around you to continue meditating when they see how it helps you.

OK, let's give it a try. First you must find a quiet place where you can sit undisturbed for 15 or 20 minutes. Sit upright with your spine straight. You can use a chair or sit against the wall. You don't have to sit Lotus, (with your legs bent in an unnatural configuration). Find a comfortable position, but not lying down. You could become so relaxed that you will fall asleep. That is not your goal. You may prefer a dark room.

Take a few very deep breaths. Hold them a few seconds and let them out slowly. Concentrate on your breathing and nothing else. This will help relax you and you will begin to feel the tension leaving your body. After a few deep breaths, let your breath come naturally.

You must choose a mantra, a one syllable word, and repeat it slowly to yourself. You can say, "Love, peace, one, God" - anything you please. Let your mind clear. If thoughts begin to take you away, come back to your mantra. With practice you will be able to let the thoughts float by. Do not let them fill your mind. It's tough but you will get it eventually. Even in the beginning you will see benefits to continuing. It is a wonderful experience. You can get addicted.

Try to meditate a few minutes at first and work your way up to 20 or 30 minutes once or twice a day. It can be very helpful if you wake up during the night and are worried or frightened. Stay in a reclined position and try to meditate. You should drift back to sleep in a few minutes. It is a very effective way to gain control over your body and mind at a time when it is out of control. Meditation can be learned from books, but it is always better to find an instructor and class to join. Try it at home and if you think you need more help, try the health food store, or the YMCA. Look for holistic doctors and practitioners in the phone book.

Guided Imagery (Visualization). There are many books written on this subject and so much to say that it is difficult to summarize for you. We practice visualization regularly because it works. You can control to a great extent what happens to your body. You may not realize your inner potential.

> "Of the 54 heart surgery patients included in a study done at Carnegie-Mellon University, **the optimists healed faster..."**

To illustrate this point, a physiologist discussing this issue in an ovarian cancer group meeting shocked the audience with the following example. She had been treating many multiple personalities over the years and discovered something quite remarkable. In many cases she would find that one personality would have diabetes or asthma, and the other personalities were well. What an outstanding example of the power of the mind! One can imagine they have an illness, but to clinically go from diabetic to healthy in the blink of the psyche is amazing. What incredible power the brain must possess.

Relate that to a visual image, and see yourself well. Perhaps it is seeing little critters inside of you nibbling away at your cancer, or seeing the radiation or chemo as healthy rays of energy burning away the disease like the sun would burn off the fog. It may be your practice visualizing yourself on a beautiful sunny beach, healthy and well. You can see yourself ten years from now with your family grown. All are forms of visualization.

All can be very powerful stimuli to your body. Dr. Bernie S. Siegel has a tape "Healing Meditations" that guides you through imagery of a healthy mind and body. We both have used it and know his tapes work.

Stop what you are doing right now.

You must choose a mantra.

Close your eyes and take a few deep breaths, let them out slowly. See good, healthful things.

Some ideas to get you started:

See God touching your shoulder and walking with you. Ask him to make you well.

Picture yourself happy and healthy surrounded by your friends and family.

Imagine your treatments working like magic zapping the cancer. See your killer T-cells working all day and night to get you healthy again and see yourself as having been successful.

Visualize animals, fish, birds, the FBI, space aliens or whomever you want, eating and destroying all cancer cells.

Pick a warm and fuzzy image or an army of tiny soldiers. It is totally up to you.

I used to call my cancer sharks out to do their duty. They roamed my tummy and ate the cancer. I even named them. Killer was the big guy. He ate every bad cell he could find. Plato ran the guard duty. He patrolled, circling and watching for any renegade cells that were looking to cause trouble. His job was to call Killer if he encountered the enemy. It sounds silly, but I felt I was doing something to help out and my sharks were taking care of me even when I was too weak or tired to concentrate. Now I visualize little white happy faces coming out of my bones, like a tiny smiling army, eating up the bad guys. — Rose

Our best recommendation is the strong suggestion that you give it a try. You can learn to do this at home from books or just on your own. Libraries and bookstores offer a great selection on visualization techniques. We have a few suggestions in the appendix.

Combining these mental exercises with body movement, is the second vitally important part of your immune boosting exercise program.

Yoga, an ancient eastern science and philosophy, is designed to bring one in union with the soul. Yoga principles are over 2000 years old. Yoga focuses on the health of the body as a whole. Its application here is that it positions each individual part of your body correctly so that it may function at its optimum potential. It is a partnership between your mind and body.

Yoga is a series of rhythmic, balanced movements. Its graceful positions appear to

Lying on cross bolster pillows

Having support under your chest makes breathing easier. This is so good for your system. You can feel your chest opening and your breath deepening with each inhalation and exhalation.

1.   Lay a bolster pillow or rolled blanket on the floor. Lay another bolster lengthwise across it. Sit on the front of the top pillow and lie back over it with your shoulders on the floor. Place a folded blanket under the head if needed. If your back is not comfortable, slide a little up or down and find a comfy position.

Stretch your legs away from your torso, and then relax them. Put your arms over your head and then relax them also. Stay in this position for 5 to 15 minutes, breathing evenly.

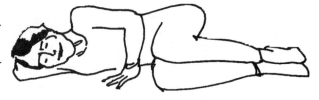

2.   To avoid straining your back when geting up, roll onto one side and get up slowly.

be artistic serene poses. Yoga will help to release tension and stretches the spine. Flexibility will give you energy and help you feel good all over. A healthy body is in a state of balance and all systems are equally supporting the others. Yoga will help you gain control of your body and any functions that may be out of balance. Each position should be comfortable or don't do it.

Positions can be relaxing, stimulating, soothing, and build concentration. Yoga is an exercise whose therapeutic value increases with practice. It helps to maintain youthful flexibility and mind/body peace. You should begin with simple positions, and as your strength increases, so do your cycles of postures.

Check with your doctor and take these precautions before you begin:

Don't wear tight clothes.

Don't practice in direct sunlight or a cold room.

Wait 4 hours after a big meal, 2 hours after eating light.

Do not hold your breath during the postures; it causes strain.

Don't force your body beyond its normal range of motion.

If you are pregnant, get expert advise from your doctor and a yoga instructor before you begin. It could be dangerous for the infant.

Yoga will leave you feeling flexible and peaceful. The postures are toning and very little movement is required. They are great when you do not feeling like hopping around the gym in your leotard.

Yoga can be learned from a book;

however it is best to locate a class.

Your spouse/family members suffer through your illness with you. Relaxation techniques are helpful to them also. If you do them together it is rewarding for both of you. *Get them involved.*

Let's talk about getting up out of the chair and moving around. This might start with a stroll around the house or yard. We know how crummy you can feel, but you will feel better if you get up and get moving.

You may need some physical therapy following surgery or after an extended period of illness.

If you feel you do, look for a progressive therapist or clinic that has worked with cancer patients before. In fact, ask if they have treated patients with your particular needs. If you feel you can start moving around a little, and the doctors give the O.K., begin.

You can start by just wiggling the fingers and rotating the wrists. Work your way around your body with gentle movements. Don't think that just taking a few steps more each day won't make any difference. *It does.* You can work your way up to a brisk walk or even some heart-pumping exercise. Walk around a park and get visual stimulation from the scenery. Set your walking routine to suit your condition. Remember: exercise is one of the best preventative remedies for fighting illness.

"How much" is good for you will depend on your physical condition. **Please ask your doctor if you can begin a program before you do any physical activity.**

Why is it important to get some kind of exercise each day?

Let's start with some very basics. Decreased muscle activity causes muscle loss. Muscles burn fat. If muscle mass decreases so does your metabolism. Your metabolic function is the chemical process that sustains your life. That means you are not functioning at an optimum level, making it harder for your systems to do their job.

On the other hand if you exercise, you stimulate the circulatory and lymphatic system as well. The lymph system, which is located mainly in the arms and legs, filters toxins, which you are full of from your cancer and its treatment, from your blood and tries to excrete them through the skin, urine or colon. The lymph system has no pumping mechanism. If you do not move those arms and legs your lymph system has a difficult time getting rid of the build-up.

Obviously the circulatory system is important in keeping nutrients and oxygen flowing normally to all tissues and cells of the body and getting rid of dead cancer cells. Without this freshening process you would die very quickly.

Exercise also builds the lungs and strengthens the heart. This is all good news. You can start immediately to help your body fight off your cancer. Certainly sounds like something you should be doing, doesn't it? The right time to begin is now, providing you have medical clearance from your doctors.

Remember:

Proceed with caution and at your own pace. Each day you can do a little more, even if it is only one or two more steps. You set the pace.

Ann Frahm, in her book, "Cancer Battle Plan", *(another must read)* started exercising after the doctors had written her off. You can bet she paced herself. Pick up her book and see how she worked through a "terminal diagnosis" and over five years later runs a retreat helping other cancer patients detoxify mind and body.

When I came home from the hospital after surgery, I couldn't even walk around the bed without help. Each day I took a few more steps and finally made it out to the bottom of the driveway. I shuffled down the street looking pretty worn out, but I was rejoicing inside. I was on my way back to my old self. I was determined to regain my energy. It worked. — Rose

---

Fresh air is one of the nicest components of your exercise program. Try to get out of the house, weather and health permitting. There is nothing like a few deep breaths of fresh air to invigorate the body and soul. Freshly-oxygenated blood flows through your body, freeing toxic blockages. Your muscles need O_2 to function properly. Give them a daily dose. They will show you their gratitude in how you feel. Put a few deep breaths on the top of your list of daily "To Do's". If you can't get out of the house, open a window. Try breathing in through your nose, holding it for a few seconds, and exhaling by pushing the air out with your tummy muscles.

> *Put a few deep breaths on the top of your list of daily "To Do's".*

I craved fresh air when I was confined to the hospital for weeks on end. One day my husband and I badgered the nurses into letting me go outside for a short vacation of fresh air. The trip to the great outdoors involved getting dressed into warm clothing (a major project), putting my IV infuser on battery pack, wearing a mask, covering my naked head with a ski cap, going down 8 floors, walking through a few halls of staring hospital guests and through the packed hospital cafeteria to gain access to the outdoor patio. Those wonderful lungfulls of fresh air, and the warm sunshine in the crisp winter air was worth every bit of the effort. I felt rejuvenated! — Shirley

If you are weak or tired from surgery or treatments, just do a little something. For an energy boost try tensing and relaxing the muscles in your feet and toes and slowly working up the body. Take a couple of deep breaths and tense and release muscles. It's a quick fix and you don't even have to get up out of your chair. Play some stimulating music. It definitely has an effect on your mood. It can be soothing or energizing, depending on how you want to feel. If it can soothe the savage beast, it can do wonders for you.

Relaxation is a great form of exercise too. A great 2-minute relaxing idea comes from Joan Borysenko's book, "Minding the Body, Mending the Mind". It will bring a quick change in physiology and attitude.

In her book Joan suggests that you shift to abdominal breathing. Abdominal breathing is the direct opposite of your day-time routine. Breathe in expanding your tummy, let it out, contract your stomach muscles. Relax as you breathe. Feel tension leave your body. In fact, slow concentrated breathing not only releases tension, but also helps to oxygenate your blood.

Get a daily dose of sunshine.

Sunlight can increase seratonin levels. Seratonin can increase energy. Melatonin is also produced which induces restful sleep. If you can't get out because of your health or the weather, then sit by a sunny window. Be careful not to over do it because too much sun can be hazardous if you are in treatment. A few minutes a day is nice.

Muscles can atrophy, or shrivel, with just a little time off your feet. Try to keep your joints and muscles as flexible as possible. You have enough to worry about without getting stiff and immobile. Simple moves done right in a chair can help out. Wiggle your toes, make circles with your feet to loosen ankles. Lift knees, bend elbows, just move around whatever and however you can.

If you are feeling well enough, get into a regular exercise routine. With approval from your doctor, start immediately. You will gain strength and flexibility quickly. Hearty exercise sends a message to the pituitary gland to release endorphins that soothe pain and make you feel happy all over. You can choose walking, bicycling, swimming, tennis, aerobics, jazzercize, anything that will get the blood flowing and heart beating.

A trip to the gym to join an aerobics class can make you feel like you have two left feet when you are well, not to mention when you are not so well. Keeping up with the perky little aerobics teachers and their ever-changing arm, leg, and hip-swinging movements is a real project for the healthy.

So, in response to demand, we have created an exercise regimen that is perfect for all participants:

EUC (pronounced 'Yuck')

EUC, or **Exercises Unencumbered by Coordination**, can be performed any time of the day or night, anywhere in the world, and to any kind of music including self-hummed stuff. You can turn on the radio, stereo or

belt out a show tune. You need not be in sync with the music. You need no special equipment or clothing. In fact, they are really funny if you do them nude, in front of a mirror.

EUCs are a series of unstructured movements set to a beat of your choice. The twist is a nice way to start. You can throw in ungraceful ballet steps, the boogaloo, a high school cheer, or just a rhythmic shuffle. Wave your arms, wiggle your butt, dance, strike a pose — who cares, just keep moving. Time will fly by if you are truly zany. A word of caution: "Don't let too many people see you doing these. There may be some question as to your mental state."

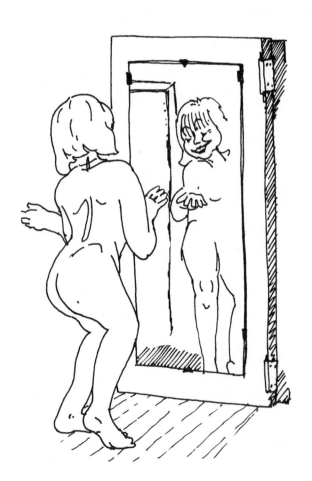

I stand in front of a full-length mirror in my underwear and watch all the flowing movement of my cushy padded thighs and derriere. I never realized what an awful dancer I was until I saw myself doing the EUCs in the mirror. No wonder my mother gave up on ballet class for me! — Rose

EUCs accomplish two things. The first is that you are getting some great exercise, which you design yourself and do at your pace in the privacy of your home. The second benefit of EUCs is that they are so silly looking and feeling that you should get a hearty laugh out of them.

Laughing is definitely therapeutic. A hearty laugh or two increases blood circulation, works the tummy muscles, and increases heart rate. It replenishes your lungs with fresh air and drops your blood pressure to a healthier level than before the uproar. Dr. Lee S. Berk at Loma Linda School of Public Health in California found that laughter had an effect on the immune and neuroendocrine systems. The study showed that an hour of laughing lowers levels of stress hormones and increase the activity of T-Cells and antibodies. Now you're talking *fun exercises.* Check the appendix for Laughter Therapy. You can view a free Candid Camera tape just for the asking.

Whatever exercises you choose to do, try to create a regular routine. Every extra movement you do daily will be healthful to you. When you first wake up in the morning, take a few deep breaths. If you feel well enough, raise your arms up over your head to gently stretch the rib cage. Focus on your breathing and try to breathe in through your nose and pull the air up from your tummy to exhale. Don't stretch too hard first thing out of bed, your muscles may be stiff from sleep.

Just move around a bit. You may find a warm shower relaxes your muscles. The warm water causes dilation of blood vessels, increasing flow to muscles and other body organs. Shower heads with massage settings and whirlpools can do wonders for relaxing muscles.

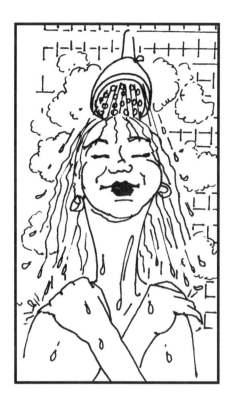

You know by now that cancer tries to take over your life, every aspect of it. Exercise will put you closer to the control button. It is a great feeling to be in charge.

The following work sheets will help you keep track of daily nutrition and exercise. Make many copies and use them every day. You'll be able to look back and see how well you have progressed.

I used to get nervous and upset because I was feeling so achy and everyone around me was healthy. I felt like I was going to scream with frustration. I would jump in the shower and let the warm water relax me. I know you're supposed to conserve water, but I stayed in there for a very long time. I came out calm and ready to continue my daily battle to get rid of the cancer. — Rose

---

nutrition
prescription

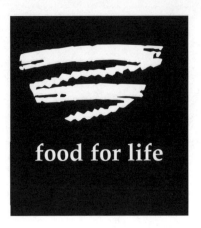

food for life

Check List

~~~ Foods I need to eat daily *(Keep this list the same unless you make a change based on good nutritional knowledge.)*

~~~ What did I forget yesterday?

~~~ How did I do today?

      Breakfast:

      Lunch:

      Dinner:

      In - between munchies:

~~~ What do I need to do tomorrow that I missed today?

motion quotient

keep on truckin'

My Daily Exercise & Activity Formula

Stand up straight. Don't give your body the wrong signals about your health. Your mind needs to send out positive vibes. Put your shoulders back, take a few slow, deep breaths and assume the position of a fighter.

The doctor said it was O.K. to do:

What type of activity?

What time(s) of Day?

How long, or how many times?

What part of the body got the workout?

How did I feel before and after?

What will I do tomorrow to make it even better?

10 ways to a beautiful day

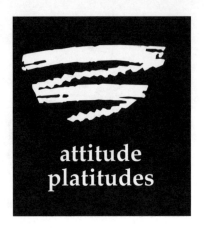

attitude platitudes

Use some of our suggestions, then think of your own. Put a sheet of paper up on the fridge or next to your bed each day and think of ways to make each day a wonderful experience. When you have them written down, try them out.

~~~ Count my blessings!

~~~ Call someone I love and tell him or her so!

~~~ Take a walk, breath some fresh air, get my blood flowing!

~~~ Listen to my favorite music!

~~~ Treat myself to some chocolate!

~~~ Get a facial!

~~~ Get into some comfy clothes and watch a great movie!

Strategy #7: Keep Financial, Insurance and Legal Concerns in Check

Fighting cancer involves more than chemotherapy and radiation. It involves paperwork and telephone calls. You will find yourself dealing with some very basic problems which can be hard to manage when you are feeling ill. But managing the medical bills, insurance forms and insurance problems, legal considerations, financial stresses and other paperwork associated with illness is important. It can also be quite time-consuming. What we offer in this chapter is information and guidelines for handling these issues, thereby easing these particular burdens for you as much as possible.

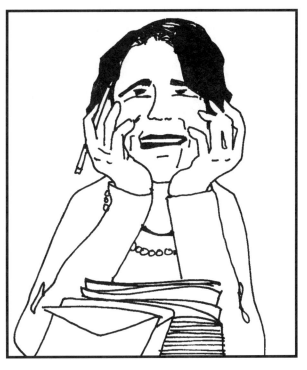

Our first bit of advice is: if you are terribly ill, try to find someone else to take care of these details for you. When you are exhausted, taking strong medications, or feeling physically ill, handling even routine financial and insurance issues can be overwhelming. We hope that you have a family member or close friend who will take over this duty for you for a while. But if not, the following information should help you handle the situation with as little effort as possible. If you have to put some of this off for a little while until you regain your strength, go ahead. *Just don't let it get too out of control.*

Medical Insurance

The best way to ensure that you have adequate medical insurance coverage for cancer treatment is to ask a variety of insurance planners about their payment policies for cancer treatment *before* you select a plan. If you did that, had a choice among plans, and were able to pick the plan with the best possible coverage, then you don't need to read the next few pages. However, few of us plan to get cancer, and most of us do not have a wide choice in insurance policies, or we simply assume that our insurer will just naturally cover our treatment costs if we become seriously ill. *Cancer is a reality check in so many ways!*

There are three basic types of health insurance:

Indemnity, Preferred Provider Organization or Network (PPO) and Health Maintenance Organization (HMO). A fourth type of insurance plan, Point of Service (POS) is fairly new, and gaining in popularity.

Each type of plan differs in areas of access to care, covered benefits, coinsurance /copayments, and claim submission procedures. There is a great deal of upheaval taking place today in the U.S. healthcare industry.

At one end of the issue spectrum is HMO's with emphasis on cost containment. Some HMO plans have a compensation system known as "capitation" wherein doctors receive a set fee for each HMO member patient. The doctor is responsible for any costs exceeding this set fee figure. Doctors are under pressure to stick to their budget, which is not a problem with healthy patients, but becomes difficult with sick patients who "erode the profit margin".

And while the traditional fee - for - service indemnity insurance, at the other end of the spectrum, offers more flexibility for the patient and the doctor, these plans are far from perfect. With no cost "cap", unscrupulous doctors can take advantage of the system. While hopefully avoiding making any kind of preferential judgment, we offer a brief description of the four major types of insurance plans.

Indemnity plans offer the most flexibility with the ability to choose any provider of services, choice of deductibles, and coinsurance. Providers submitting claims are paid benefits on a reasonable and customary basis. Indemnity plans suffer from rising costs and inability to maintain those costs.

PPO plans have two parts. The company, which develops the benefits, provides administration and pays the claims and the contracted providers who submit the claims. The company contracts with the providers for each category of services, establishing a maximum cost; i.e. the rates are pre-determined by contract. As with Indemnity, you have a deductible and copayment percentage. Your choice of doctor, hospital and other providers is limited to those providers who are contracted with the plan. The selection is usually large. The choice of physicians, hospitals and other providers contracted with the plan is open at all times. If necessary, non-network providers may also be used.

HMO's are also composed of two separate parts: the plan and the providers. The providers are contracted by the plan to provide services for out- and in-patient services. Fees are pre-established by contract, with the doctors and medical groups assuming some of the risk in costs of services. The plan's goal is to provide adequate services while containing medical costs. These plans, while offering more benefits and lower costs, limit your choice of providers and offer a more systematized form of care. You also need approval to see a specialist, which can cause difficulty when seeking to obtain the best possible treatment for your cancer.

Point of Service plans are the latest type of insurance plan to become popular, combining the features of HMO and PPO insurance. You can choose a primary care physician for the HMO benefits part of the plan, while having access to contracted PPO and non-network physicians. The cost of these plans is 10 to 20% higher than a traditional HMO.

According to information provided to patients and their families by The Association of Community Centers, there are certain minimum standards for cancer benefits in insurance policies that we should all be aware of, including;

✘ Coverage for all cancer-related drugs and therapies that are FDA approved and selected by a physician.

✘ Coverage for new procedures, drugs and technologies that have been established by scientific literature. New technologies are considered to be standard therapy when scientific research clearly demonstrates their effectiveness in treating cancer. In case of confusion about what is considered "standard therapy", there should be a policy provision that requires the insurer to contact a state association of cancer specialists or a chapter of the Association of Community Cancer Centers for an evaluation of the therapy in question.

✘ Coverage should not be denied on the basis that a drug was used in combination with other drugs. Many standard cancer drug treatment protocols involve the administration of more than one drug at a time.

✘ Coverage should include special payment status for drugs designated as Group 'C' Agents by the NCI, and drugs granted 'Treatment IND' status by the FDA.

✘ Coverage should include payment for standard patient care costs associated with patients enrolled in clinical trials approved by the FDA and N.I.H. agencies.

The public, hospitals, doctors, nurses, employers and insurance companies are all concerned with controlling healthcare costs. Unfortunately, in the quest to control costs, some insurance companies are denying payment for new, effective cancer therapies. They have their reasons, which are of small consolation to you if you need the treatment.

Sometimes the insurance company is not aware of the new treatment and therefore refuses to pay. If this is your case, make sure your doctor, hospital or cancer center provides your insurer with information about the effectiveness of the new treatment and ask for an appeal of their decision to deny. A letter from your physician explaining the reason for and importance of a certain medication or treatment may tip the scale in your favor. Some insurance companies, in their quest to control costs, limit the selection of drugs. In a further attempt to lower their costs, they may try to limit your doctor's selection of therapies to those that are low in cost. This can force you to undergo older, less adequate treatment in lieu of the most effective, state-of-the-art treatment available. *Appeal! You are entitled to the best.*

Some insurers are restricting payment to only those uses initially approved by the FDA. However, after the FDA's initial review of a drug, doctors and scientists continue to find new, effective uses for approved drugs in treating a number of types of cancers that are not included on the FDA label. Although these new uses get reviewed and listed in three major drug reference books that are recognized by the

U.S. Congress, some insurance companies are still restricting payment to only the original uses. Appeals are always worth the small amount of time and effort it takes to file one, although a decision reversal is not likely. In addition, some insurers are not paying for medical costs related to Clinical Trials. The National Cancer Institute, the National Institutes of Health and the FDA conduct research studies of investigational cancer therapies, providing patients with access to promising new treatments that have not yet been approved by the FDA for wide-spread use. The manufacturers of investigational agents often provide drugs free of charge to patients on research studies. Unfortunately, many insurers refuse to pay for "standard" treatments associated with these studies, including hospital stays, office visit, lab tests and drugs.

What can you do if payment is denied?

Your doctor can provide your insurance company with the results of scientific studies that prove a particular drug is effective treatment for your cancer. Also, the staff at your hospital or cancer center will provide your insurer with information to obtain payment for hospital stays, lab tests, etc. Usually this is sufficient to rectify the problem and the claim is paid.

However, if these efforts fail, your doctor and the other professionals involved with your care can obtain assistance from a number of reimbursement specialists who operate hotlines for various drug manufacturers. These specialists provide an array of services, including literature searches of pertinent studies and direct contacts with involved insurers. In some states, cancer

doctors have formed organization that are actively involved in educating the decision makers at the insurance companies about effective new treatments, and are also working with cancer patient advocacy groups to pass state laws that require insurers to meet minimum standards of coverage.

As a last resort, you can sue your insurance company to obtain payment for treatment. There is no guarantee, of course, that the courts will side with you, but the legal route is one to considerate if all other efforts fail.

What to do if care is denied?

Doctors, lawyers and consumer advocates suggest the following:

✗ Know your schedule of benefits. If you have questions, call your member service department or your company's insurance plan supervisor.

✗ Work with your doctor. Ideally, your doctor should be your advocate. Enlist his help in procuring approval for the treatment. If your doctor will not work with you to gain permission for treatment, find another physician, one who will support you. (If you are an HMO member, check your benefits brochure to see when you are allowed to switch doctors.

Some plans are restrictive, allowing you to change only once a year). If a treatment is denied by insurance, find out why. See an outside specialist who is willing to write a letter to your insurer explaining the need for the treatment. Forward the letter to the president of the insurance company, if needed.

Some hospital and doctor bills are laundry lists of injections, fluids, therapies, etc. One of my surgery bills was so confusing it took me several tries to figure it out. When I did, I noticed that line items that were months old were not being paid, but more recent charges were. After much ado from the insurance company it was discovered that the hospital had never called for authorization and the insurance refused to pay. This was the hospital's fault and they credited several thousand dollars off my bill. It pays to check them over. — Rose

---

✘ Appeal the decision by submitting a written request for treatment. Appeals can be lengthy, so be prepared for this process to take a while, and there is no guarantee of success – so be ready to go the distance.

✘ File a grievance with your insurer's grievance committee. If your insurer's grievance committee is an independent panel, you stand a better chance of success. Otherwise, it may be somewhat like asking Dad after Mom said no!

✘ Contact your state insurance commission. It may intervene if your insurer is clearly in the wrong.

✘ Contact a consumer advocate group, which may offer time-saving tips and put you in contact with other patients. Groups have more clout than individuals.

✘ Consult a lawyer. A lawyer's carefully worded letter sometimes can prod an insurer into providing coverage. Insurance companies don't like the adverse publicity of a potential lawsuit.

Pre-existing conditions:

On August 22, 1996, President Clinton signed the Kennedy-Kassebaum Bill, which is also known as the Health Insurance Portability and Accountability Act of 1996. This bill calls for limits on pre-existing condition exclusions in insurance policies.

Insurers may not impose pre-existing condition exclusions or deny coverage for more than 12 months for any condition that was diagnosed or treated in the proceeding six months.

This is an important step in the right direction for cancer patients and survivors. Although it is only a small step, we herald any action that improves our rights to equality under the law.

✘ Pay for the treatment yourself. Never do without life-saving treatment because of insurance problems. Once you have saved your life, then you can fight the insurance company for proper compensation!

Financial Assistance

Cancer imposes a heavy economic burden on both you and your family. If you have medical insurance, your health plan will pay for part of your medical care. But depending on the extent and type of cancer treatment you receive and the type of insurance you have, your share of the expenses can be an amazingly large sum of money! Unless you are quite wealthy, you can pretty much count on the fact that battling cancer is not only going to alter you physically, emotionally, and psychologically, but also financially. But as with all the other aspects of this disease, there are people and agencies available to help you.

If you do not have medical insurance coverage, or if you do but are not able to cover all the costs of your care, there are numerous resources available to help, including but not limited to government-sponsored programs and services provided by voluntary organizations. You need to discuss any concerns you may have regarding the cost of your care with your physicians, the hospital/clinic business office, and/or the medical social worker.

Resources which may offer assistance:

✗ Cancer Information Service (CIS), a program of the National Cancer Institute, is an excellent first step in looking for financial assistance resources. The information specialists at CIS have extensive training in providing up-to-date and understandable information. They can answer questions in English and Spanish and can send free printed material. The CIS office, which services your geographic area, can offer you specific information about many cancer-related services and resources available to you. Call CIS at 1-800-4-CANCER (1-800-422-6237) for information and the telephone number of the office nearest you.

✗ Social Security provides income for eligible elderly and disabled individuals. Call the Social Security Administration (SSA) at 1-800-SSA-1213 to receive information on eligibility and explanation of coverage, or to apply for benefits.

✗ Supplemental Security Income (SSI) supplements Social Security payments for those individuals who meet certain income and asset criteria. SSI is administered by the Social Security Administration. Call SSA at 1-800-SSA-1213 (1-800-772-1213) for information on eligibility, for explanation of coverage, or to apply.

✗ Medicare is a Federal health insurance program for those people who receive Social Security benefits (including people who are 65 or older, people of any age with permanent kidney failure, and disabled people under age 65 who have been receiving Social Security payments for at least 24 months). For information on eligibility, explanations of coverage, or to apply, call 1-800-SSA-1213.

✗ Medicaid (Medical Assistance) provides health insurance for low-income and indigent people who are elderly, blind, or disabled, as well as for the certain groups of children. Contact your local Department of Social Services or the SSA.

✗ **General Assistance** programs provide housing, food, prescription medications and other medical expenses for those who are not eligible for other programs. Funds for General Assistance programs are often limited. For further information, contact your local Dept. of Social Services.

✗ **Veteran's Benefits** are available to eligible veterans and their dependents at VA Medical Centers. Treatment for service-connected conditions is provided and treatment for other conditions may be available based on the veteran's financial need. For information, call 1-800-827-1000.

✗ **Hill-Burton** is a program through which hospitals receive construction funds from the Federal Government. Hospitals receiving these funds are required to provide some services to people who cannot afford to pay for their hospitalization. To obtain a list of Hill-Burton hospitals in your area, or to get information about eligibility, call 1-800-638-0742.

✗ **The American Cancer Society (ACS)** office serving your area may offer reimbursement for expenses related to your cancer treatment. These may include reimbursement for medicine and/or medical supplies, and transportation costs (usually only ground transportation

expenses). Call 1-800-ACS-2345 for the telephone number of the ACS serving you, or check the white pages of your telephone directory under American Cancer Society.

✗ **The Leukemia Society of America (LSA)** offers information and financial aid to parties who have leukemia, non-Hodgkin's lymphoma, Hodgkin's disease, or multiple myeloma. Call 1-800-955-4LSA to request the society's booklet describing LSA's Patient Aid Program or the telephone number of your local LSA office.

✗ **Patient Assistance Programs** are offered by some pharmaceutical manufacturers to help patients pay for drugs. Talk with your physician or medical social worker to learn whether any of your medications may be available at reduced cost through such a program. For a complete and updated list of drug manufacturer's offering programs, call the U. S. Senate Department of Aging at (202) 224-5364, or access OncoLink on the Internet at http://oncolink.upenn.edu. The list is free.

✗ **Service Organizations and Community Voluntary Agencies** may offer help. Contact the Salvation Army, Lutheran Social Services, Jewish Social Services, Catholic Charities, the Lions Club, and other organizations to see if help is available. Check your local phone directory's yellow pages under Clubs, Social Service Organizations, Religious

Organizations for organizations that may be able to offer assistance.

✖ **Churches and Synagogues** may provide financial help or services to their members. If you need help, talk to your clergy person.

✖ **NPATH, the National Patient Air Transport Hotline**, offers assistance with air transportation. Contact NPATH at 1-800-296-1217. **Air Alliance** is a nationwide association of humanitarian flying organizations dedicated to community service. Using their own time and general aviation aircraft, pilot members of these organizations help hundreds of people every month travel to facilities where they are able to receive medical attention they need. There is no charge for their service. Other organizations which offer similar air transportation service are **Air Life Line** at 1-800-446-1231, **Air-Evac International, Inc** at 1-800-982-5806, and **Corporate Angels Network** at (914) 328-1313). If you must fly commercially, contact the airline and be candid with them. Some airlines offer reduced fares for patients going for treatment.

Sources of Income from One's Own Assets:

✖ **Reverse Mortgages**, which are sponsored by the U.S. Department of Housing and Urban Development, can provide cash to terminally ill patients over 62 years of age who have equity in their home.

✖ **Private Loans**, made by close friends and relatives who might not otherwise be able to make a private loan, but who do have equity in their homes and are over 62 can also use the reverse mortgage technique, paying off the mortgage with the proceeds of your life insurance policy. A private loan avoids discounting that occurs in a Viatical Settlement (see below) and are not taxable to you as income, nor do they count for eligibility by SSI. Medicaid, and some other sources of financial assistance.

✖ **Life Insurance Policies** offer several means of obtaining necessary cash to improve the quality of a patient's life. This in turn can add to the length of your life. In addition to the above mentioned techniques of private loans and reverse mortgages based on eventual repayment from the insurance policy, there is a new and complicated, but increasingly more common technique - a **Viatical Settlement**.

✖ **Viatication**, derived from the Latin word viaticum meaning "provision for the journey". Before we explain this source of finances further, we wish to point out that this is an option for terminally ill patients with a limited life expectancy. Because it can give the terminally ill patient money needed to provide financial help, which can promote physical health and prolong one's lifespan, we wanted to include it. However, we hope that this is not an option you need to consider.

The viatication of your insurance policy is the sale of the policy to a viatical settlement firm at a discounted value.

The process is more complicated than we wish to go into in this publication, but we will give you a brief synopsis of the process. The patient sells his or her life insurance policy to a company specializing in such purchases. There are approximately 54 such firms in business today, and the field is growing. These firms are sensitive to the needs and rights of the terminally ill.

Their clients are instructed to secure the advice of legal counsel, accountants and/or their financial planners, and any health or social service agency who is helping the patient with financial assistance. Written releases and consent documents from formerly named beneficiaries and heirs, relatives, and interested parties are required, as well as eligibility determination by medical professionals. Confidentiality is guaranteed to all involved parties, a reconsideration period is included, after which qualifying insurance policies are purchased through a legal trust or escrow arrangement. Firms retain their own legal counsel, of course, to handle compliance issues, policies, and document preparation. A major hurdle in viatical settlements is valuation of the policy. This involves several factors: face amount of the policy, cash loans, premium expenses, costs of financing, the person's life expectancy, and legal, medical and administrative costs, together with the nature of policy provision of group based policies.

These viatical settlements can be a viable form of income for patients who need money to improve the quality of their lives, and pay for care. However, they are limited to the "definitively terminally ill". Additionally, receiving insurance money makes you ineligible for SSI, Medicaid, welfare, food stamps, and housing assistance. Also, the benefits are subject to Income Tax. Congress is now

For information on Viatical Settlements: contact the:

National Viatical Association
7910 Woodmont Avenue, Suite 1430, Bethesda, MD 20814

The Viatical Association of America
1200 19th Street, N.W., Suite 300 Washington, DC 20036

your **State Attorney General**, or your **State Insurance Commissioner**

The Federal Trade Commission publishes an excellent *FREE* pamphlet explaining viaticals.
Call (202) 326-2222;
or for TDD, call (202) 326-2502.
For on-line Internet access, find the FTC at consumer.ftc.gov or http://www.ftc.gov.

considering exempting both viaticals and accelerated death benefits from income tax, but as of the printing of this book, income tax was still payable on these benefits.

✘ **Accelerated Benefits** riders on insurance offer another option worthy of consideration if medical proof of impending death (usually six months or less) can be provided to the insurance company. With this program, you (the insured-owner) receive all or part of the death benefit at some discount of the face amount, with remainder going to your beneficiaries.

✘ **Transfer of Ownership** is yet another means for getting cash from your insurance. The new owner - a trusted friend - can then accelerate or viaticate the policy based on your limited life expectancy.

The disadvantage of attaining funds from your life insurance policy is that these programs are based on your "limited life expectancy", which falls in the face of all we believe in, "Hope, Knowledge, and Survival". But we would be remiss if we did not offer you this information, as it may be necessary for you to make use of one of these resources in order to improve the quality of your life and your medical care.

Income Tax Information:

Keeping track of your medical expenses is important. Medical costs that are not covered by your insurance policy(ies) may be deductible from your annual income before taxes. Expenses such as mileage for trips to and from medical appointments, out-of-pocket costs for treatment, prescription drugs or equipment, the cost of meals during lengthy medical visits, and parking expenses may be deductible.

Keeping Accurate Records:

At the end of this chapter there are two worksheets. One is a list of the records and receipts you need to keep while you are undergoing treatment. It is really difficult to think about these practical matters while you are feeling ill, so if you can pawn this off on a loved one, please do.

Most of us don't realize until income tax time that many of the expenses of cancer treatment which are not covered by medical insurance (parking, travel expenses including mileage, etc.) are part of your medical expense deductions. (The second worksheet is a copy of a Living Will).

Medical Bills

The medical bills seem to arrive in your mailbox before the Get Well and Encouragement cards. And they keep coming long after your treatment is over. They can truly overwhelm you, not just with their dollar amount, but for the sheer volume of them and the incredibly confusing way they are formatted. Try to keep them organized. We realize that this may be difficult when you are feeling unwell, but if you start out with some semblance of organization, you won't be mired in paperwork later. Keep separate files or envelopes for each provider, and look over the bills as they come in. Be sure you are being billed for the proper treatment, services, etc. Hospital bills require extra scrutiny, as they usually contain numerous charges. It is not unusual to find yourself being billed for a service or medication you never received.

For each provider, have a pending file and a paid file. Mark on each bill the date the invoice was sent to your primary insurer, so you can easily refer to that if your provider calls regarding payment. Some insurers take longer to pay than others, and sometimes the provider doesn't send the bill to the insurer promptly or accurately, further delaying reimbursement. If you have a secondary insurer, you must repeat the pending process.

After your bills have been paid by your insurer(s), you can mainstream them into your own regular bill-paying system and then file them in the provider's paid file when you have impoverished yourself to pay them. We highly recommend the "one file for each provider" system, because it enables you to access all the billing info for each provider quickly and easily. Medical billing systems are confusing enough without adding to the perplexity by having to search through a pile of bills and insurance company Explanation of Benefits forms from ALL your providers to find the ones you need.

If you need help dealing with outstanding medical bills, we suggest you make arrangements to personally discuss your situation with both the hospital/clinic and the physician(s)' business offices. In many cases, hospitals and physicians are willing to work out reasonable long-term payment plans; or in the case of indigence, may be willing to negotiate a discount.

You have a lot of busy work ahead of

you just keeping the files straight. Don't let this project become overwhelming. If you don't feel like keeping your files up one week, O.K. don't. Just put all the mail next to your organized filing system and get back to it when you can.

Some days it just isn't going to get done. Unfortunately, the bills will keep coming every month. If you miss-file, or don't file, don't worry — you can do it next month with the very same bill. Do check the doctor bills. It is possible to receive bills that are not yours, for hospitals you've never been in and treatments you've never received.

The important issue is that you know that you must organize and keep up with the paperwork. Remember, you can set your own pace on getting it done; however, try to get into a routine of sorts because you can easily fall very far behind. When you are feeling better you may have to do battle to defend yourself with insurance companies, doctors, and even collection agencies. Have your paper trail easy to follow!

Employment Issues

If you feel as though your work environment is not friendly during and after your illness, you have recourse. Under Federal law (Federal Rehabilitation Act of 1973 and the Americans with Disabilities Act of 1990), most employers cannot discriminate against handicapped workers, including people with cancer. These laws apply to federal employers, employers that receive federal funds, and private companies with 15 or more employees. If you think a private employer discriminated against you because of your cancer, you should file your complaint with the closest regional office of the Equal Employment Opportunities Commission. To obtain the location of your regional EEO's office, call 800/USA-EEOC.

For more information about your legal rights, call:

✗ Your local chapter of the American Cancer Society

✗ Your State Department of Labor or Office of Civil Rights

✗ Regional office of the American Civil Liberties Union

✗ Your representative or senator

Legal Issues

The Living Will

A Living Will also referred to as an "advanced directive" is a legal document, which declares that you do not wish to be kept alive by artificial means or heroic measures. This is a recognized statement of your right to forego treatment and has been upheld in court. Legally referred to as "self-determination or autonomy", it states your desire to "go on your own terms". More than 40 states have laws allowing individuals to make these advance healthcare decisions, and a federal law was enacted in 1991 requires all publicly funded hospitals, nursing homes, and hospices to inform incoming patients of their right to make a Living Will.

Read the Living Will carefully, and adjust it to fit your situation and wishes. If you decide to sign the document, be sure to tell everyone close to you that you have one and give them copies. Sign the copies. The accessibility of your Living Will is most important. It should be kept close by, not in your safety deposit box or locked in a safe! You

need to have access at a moment's notice. We suggest that if you travel, take a copy with you. Better yet, keep a copy in your purse!

Your health care team and lawyer need to be informed and given copies, to help ensure that your wishes are carried out. If you are hospitalized, make sure a copy is put in your records. Depending upon your circumstances, you may wish to appoint someone who can make binding decisions (power of attorney) for you about medical care in the event you can no longer do so. *Choose someone you can trust to abide by your wishes, who knows your view about specific treatment or any religious considerations that need to be taken into account.*

You can obtain a copy the Living Will, in the form preferred by the state you live in, from Concern for Dying (CFD), 250 West 57th Street, New York, NY 10017, (212) 246-6962. Lawyers also have copies of Living Wills, although most will charge you for it. You may also be able to obtain a form, together with information and governing guidelines for these directives from the Attorney General's Office in your state.

We have included a sample copy of a Living Will at the end of this chapter. Please note that, according to CFD, signing a Living Will document will not adversely affect any life insurance policy you have and will not be interpreted as suicide.

Durable Power of Attorney

A Durable Power of Attorney is an advance directive, which appoints someone to make health care decisions for you if you become incapacitated, even temporarily. We recommend that you combine this document or include it with your Living Will, so that your attorney-in-fact will have guidance in making the right decisions for you.

mportant numbers to keep

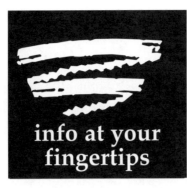

info at your fingertips

PHARMACY NAME

PHARMACIST

TELEPHONE NUMBER

DOCTOR

OFFICE MANAGER

TELEPHONE NUMBER

DOCTOR

OFFICE MANAGER

TELEPHONE NUMBER

DOCTOR

OFFICE MANAGER

TELEPHONE NUMBER

HOSPITAL   TELEPHONE NUMBER

BILLING DEPARTMENT   TELEPHONE NUMBER

ACCOUNT NUMBERS

INSURANCE COMPANY   TELEPHONE NUMBER

CUSTOMER REPRESENTATIVE

ACCOUNT NUMBER

INSURANCE COMPANY   TELEPHONE NUMBER

CUSTOMER REPRESENTATIVE

ACCOUNT NUMBER

Saving Records & Receipts

Medical Expense Records to keep for Income Tax Purposes and Bill Reconcilliation

✗ Prescription medicines & Drug Costs
✗ Physicians' and Nurses' Bills
✗ Hospital Bills
✗ Cost of Insurance Premiums
✗ Insurance Reimbursement
✗ Transportation Costs for Medical Appointments, Treatments, etc. (the IRS allows 10 cents/mile)
✗ Lodging Costs associated with Treatment, etc.
✗ Other Misc. Medical Expenses (cost for prosthetics etc.)

General Records

✗ All Medical Bills, sorted by Provider
✗ All Insurance Explanation of Benefit Forms
✗ Copies of any bills you sub mitted to insurer yourself
✗ Copies of any not-reim bursable bills (uncovered procedures or pre-deductible costs)
✗ Records of Transportation Costs
✗ Lodging Receipts
✗ Prosthetic Expenses (includ ing Wigs)
✗ Medical Supplies' Receipts (Catheter Care Kits, etc.)

You can obtain a copy of the Living Will in the form preferred by the state you live in, from :

Concern for Dying (CFD)
250 West 57th Street
New York, NY 10017
(212) 246-6962

135

LIVING WILL OF _____

       I,   (Name)   , of   (Town, State)   , request that, if my condition is deemed terminal or if I am determined to be permanently unconscious, I be allowed to die and not be kept alive through life support systems. By terminal condition I mean that I have an incurable or irreversible medical condition which, without the administration of life support systems, will, in the opinion of my attending physicians, result in death within a relatively short time. By permanently unconscious I mean that I am in a permanent coma or persistent vegetative state, which is an irreversible condition in which I am at no time aware of myself or the environment and show no behavioral response to the environment. The life support systems which I do not want include, but are not limited to:

       Artificial Respiration   (   )

       Cardiopulmonary Resuscitation   (   )

       Artificial Means of Providing Nutrition and Hydration   (   )

       (Cross out and initial life support systems you want administered.)

       I do not intend any direct taking of my life, but only that my dying not be unreasonably prolonged.

       Other specific requests:

       This request is made, after careful reflection, while I am of sound mind.

_____(Legal Signature)   (Date)

       (Name in Bold Type)

       This document was signed in our presence, by the above-named,   (Name in Type) , who appeared to be eighteen years of age or older, of sound mind and able to understand the nature and consequences of health care decisions at the time the document was signed.

_____ of _____

_____ of _____

STATE OF _____)

) ss.   (Town)   (Date)

COUNTY OF _____)

       Personally appeared   (Name in Bold Type)   , signer of the foregoing instrument, and acknowledged the same to be her free act and deed, before me.

                                              _____

                                            Commissioner of the Superior Court

                                            Notary Public

                                            My Commission Expires: (Date)

In Conclusion

In the process of research and writing this book, we learned a great deal about cancer, and more importantly, women with cancer. We found that women are much stronger than they give themselves credit for. We may feel weak while we are in the clutches of the disease and its treatment, but we learn that in truth we are tremendously strong. Fighting cancer takes power, energy, stamina and courage. The women we met possessed those traits, plus large doses of hope and faith.

We discovered that cancer often strikes with little warning and few symptoms, and that women need to learn to "read" their bodies, trust their instincts, and be informed. The more that we know about our disease and ourselves the better prepared we are to demand and receive the first-rate medical care we are entitled to.

Cancer may make changes in your life. Most people are not the same after the onset of their cancer. In their quest for survival, they come to realize that significant changes become necessary in the manner in which life is viewed. This can be manifest in jobs, diet, relationships, etc. Healing comes with a price. Pay it and go on with your life. Some cancer patients say that they view their illness as a blessing. It is difficult to see that when you are in treatment, but in time, and with retrospect, you may come to feel the same way.

Surviving patients often regard their cancer experience as an opportunity for a new life with new goals. Accept what has happened to you and let your mind and body heal and become whole again. *Let go of the old and live for the future and the new you.*

Survival is not about living forever. Survival is about quality of life and peace of mind. We want you to survive and live each day well and happy.

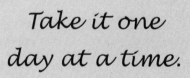

Take it one day at a time.

"We are not able to count our days, but we can make each day count."

-Unknown

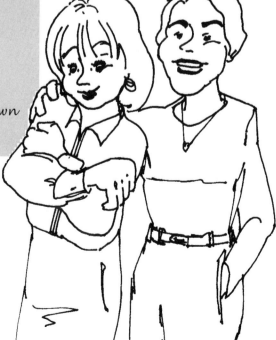

Appendix
Where to Get Cancer Information and Assistance

With a communication program, computer, and modem, people are now able to access a wealth of information about cancer that was heretofore unavailable. If you are able to take advantage of this technology, please do so. We have listed resources with telephone numbers and some of the web addresses that have cancer information on them. The number of web-sites has become so numerous as to be almost unmanageable. We will supply you here with some of the basic contacts. These addresses will lead you to others, and before you know it you will be overwhelmed with information and support.

It is important to note, however, that access to the Internet is not a necessity. In most cases, the organizations and services listed below are also accessible by telephone and/or mail, and we have provided telephone numbers and addresses whenever possible.

American Brain Tumor Association can be reached by telephone at **1-800-886-2282** or by **fax at 1-847-827-9918**. ABTA offers:

  Message Line Newsletter
  Physician Resource Listings
  Support Group Listings by State
  Connections Pen-Pal Program
  Fellowship Research Awards
  Lebow Conference on Etiology (causes)
    of Brain Tumors

ABTA Brain Tumor Symposium for
    patients, families, healthcare profes-
    sionals (next symposium is July, 1997)
Internet accessible materials
Brain Tumor Survivor's Guide to the Internet

American Cancer Society provides general information and patient services for people with cancer and their families. Information on support groups, financial assistance, and specific cancers and their treatments are available.

ACS's Reach to Recovery program has been helping women deal with breast cancer for over 25 years.

The Look Good – Feel Better program helps women undergoing radiation or chemotherapy manage the temporary skin problems and hair loss that treatment can cause. In some communities, volunteers transport patients to and from treatment. The ACS is an excellent place to start searching for information and support. Call **1-800-ACS-2345** or your local chapter listed in your telephone directory. Reach ACS on-line at HYPERLINK
http://www.cancer.org/

American Cancer Society's Breast Cancer Network offers research information and support services. Online at
http://www.cancer.org/bcnmiss.html

American Institute for Cancer Research (AICR) offers free services including information, support group lists, and a pen pal program. 1759 R. Street, NW, Washington, D.C. 20009, **1-800-843-8114** (Nutrition Hotline), **1-202-328-7744** (In Washington), **fax: 1-202-328-7226** Internet Address: AICR.ORG/AICR

American Medical Associations features an online physician finder that allows you to search the AMA's database of more than 650,000 doctors, searching by name, specialty or location. Their website is located at: http://www.ama-assn.org/

Art's Leukemia and Bone Marrow Transplant Links is a hotlist of web addresses that have cancer-related information on them. Most of the links are related to BMT and leukemia info, but there are some links to general cancer information. He provides some excellent links to information on drugs and pharmaceuticals, institutional servers, journals, papers and reports, alternative therapies, and other types of cancer. This is a good place to browse. On-line: http://rattler.cameron.edu/leukemia/index .html

Biological Therapy Institute Foundation is an information resource for patients and doctors on biopharmaceuticals in cancer therapy. P.O. Box 681700, Franklin TN 37068-1700, 1-615-790-7535, fax: 1-615-794-9110.

Bone Marrow Transplant (BMT) Newsletter publishes a bi-monthly newsletter for bone marrow transplant and stem cell transplant patients. Provides attorney referrals for insurance problems. 1985 Spruce Avenue, Highland Park, IL 60035,

1-847-831-1913, fax: 1-847-831-1943, E-mail: bmtnews@transit.nyser.net

CancerCare, Inc. based in New York City, provides assistance to people with any type of cancer, at any stage of illness. Available throughout the country, CancerCare's services are free of charge. In addition to a toll-free counseling line which offers emotional support, problem solving assistance, guidance about doctor-patient communication and second opinions, plus assistance with "finding your way" through the health care system, Cancer-Care provides referrals to other support services, educational seminars, conferences, and materials, financial assistance, and all-important information about cancer and treatment. Contact CancerCare at **1-800-813-HOPE (4673)**, or at the CancerCare Central Office, 1180 Avenue of the Americas, 2nd Floor, New York, NY 10036 or on-line at: http://www.cancercare.org email: info@cancercare.org

CancerCare OnLine Support is an on-line support group run by trained facilitators. Access is at: http://www.cancercareinc.org/onlineasst .html

CancerGuide is an information page that is dedicated to helping you find answers to your questions about cancer on the Net. From CancerGuide's homepage, you can access OncoLink, CancerNet, and Web service engines Lycos and Alta Vista. On-line: http://cancerguide.org/

Appendix / CONTINUED

CANCER HOTLINES:

Pompano Beach, FL	305-721-7600
Kansas City, MO	816-932-8453
Pittsburgh, PA	412-782-4023
Fort Worth, TX	817-535-0757
Little Rock, AR	501-375-1212
St. Louis, MO	314-962-6007

Cancer Information Service is a free service offered by the National Cancer Institute. It provides information on the latest treatments and where these treatments are available. Call **1-800-4-Cancer.**

CancerNet is an up-to-date, extensive source of information about cancer. Maintained by the National Cancer Institute (NCI), it includes a list of information sources called MEDLINE. You can contact CancerNet via e-mail: cancnet@icicb.nci.nih.gov On-line: http://icic.nci.nih.gov/ or voice telephone: **1-800-4 CANCER**

Cansearch is a guide to cancer resources on the Net, provided by the National Coalition for Cancer Survivorship. The guide offers assistance in finding sources on the Net to go to for cancer resources. On-line: http://dansearch.org/canserch/cansrch.html

CHEMOcare offers emotional support to patients and families for chemo and radiation treatments staffed by survivors. 231 North Ave. West, Westfield, NJ 07090-1428, **1-800-55-CHEMO (outside NJ), 1-908-233-1103 (inside NJ), fax: 1-908-233-0228**

The Chemotherapy Foundation supports research to develop more effective diagnosis techniques and therapies for the control and cure of cancer. Conduct educational programs for physicians and medical professionals and publishes patient information booklets. 183 Madison Avenue, #403, New York, NY. 11016, **1-212-213-9292, fax: 1-212-689-5164**

GrannyBarb's Leukemia Links offers a great deal of information about leukemia. It also offers some information of a general cancer nature. The address for Barb Lackritz's page is: http://walden.mo.net/~lackritz/index.html

Hospice offers special programs and services designed to meet the needs of terminally ill patients and families. Plans are created to provide the best quality of life for life limited patients. Hospice also provides bereavement support. Contact your local Hospice center. You can find them through the home care department of your hospital or call your local American Cancer Society for help.

International Cancer Alliance provides free information on cancer staging, treatment, diagnostic tests, and clinical trials. "Cancer Breakthroughs" is a report sent quarterly. Donations accepted, but not required. 4853 Cordell Ave, Ste. 11, Bethesda, MD 20814, **1-800-422-7361** or http://www.icare.org/icare

International Myeloma Foundation promotes, educates, and funds research for patients and doctors about myeloma. Publishes a quarterly newsletter, Myeloma Today. 2120 Stanley Hills Drive, Los Angeles, CA 90046, **1-800-452-CURE, fax: 1-213-656-1182.**

Where to Get Cancer Information and Assistance

Laughter Therapy is a private, non-profit organization founded by Allen Funt which offers a laughter therapy program to individuals with an illness. The program provides four "Candid Camera" videos compiled specifically for the Laughter Therapy program; after each video is viewed, the next one is sent, etc. until all four have been viewed. For further information and access to Laughter Therapy, write Laughter Therapy, P. O. Box 827, Monterey, CA 93942.

Living Beyond Breast Cancer, based in Narbeth, Pennsylvania, offers a 24-hour "warmline" service staffed by trained volunteers who are all breast cancer survivors. Callers are matched to a volunteer who has experienced the same treatment, i.e. mastectomy, lumpectomy, reconstruction, as the caller. Information including pamphlets, videos, outreach programs, and support are available by calling the "warmline" at **610-617-1035, or LBBC at 610-668-1320.**

Lymphoma Research Foundation of **America, Inc**. is a non-profit group that funds research grants to projects to cure lymphoma and improve treatments. They provide educational materials, free support groups and a national "buddy system" linking patients, and a quarterly newsletter. 880 Venice Blvd., #207, Los Angeles, CA 90034, **1-310-204-7040, fax:1-310-204-7043,** E-mail: HYPERLINK mailto:LRFA@aol.com LRFA@aol.com, Internet Address: http://users.aol.com/lrfa/lrfa.html

Make the Day Count publishes a newsletter. For information contact: Make the Day Count, 101142 South Union Street, Alexandria, VA 22314-3323, 314-348-1619.

Medicare Hotline, **1-800-368-5779** for information about Social Security, Disability, and Medicare.

Mediconsult.com is a free-of-charge "virtual medical clinic" which provides high quality patient-oriented medical information and moderated support to patients, their families, and health care professionals. This site offers information on many forms of cancer, plus the Cancer Emotional Support Group, moderated by Dr. Jeff Kane. Access at: http://www.mediconsult.com/

Medscape is a membership service (no fee). Upon registration, you choose an ID and password, Once you have received a usable ID and password, you have access to the Medscape's many resources. Medscape's on-line address is: http://www.medscape.com

Medsite is a medical search engine that allows you to do keyword searches to locate the best medical sites online. An excellent first online stop, Medsite is at: http://www.medsite.com/

National Alliance of Breast Cancer **Organizations** (NABCO) is a network of breast cancer organizations, which provides information, assistance and referral to anyone who has questions about breast cancer. The network also serves as a voice for the interests and concerns of breast cancer survivors and women at risk. Call: **1- 212-889-0606** or write at NABCO, 9 East 37th Street, 10th Floor, New York, NY 10006.

National Coalition for Cancer Survivorship is an organization that provides information about survivor groups across the country. It also offers "Living Through Cancer: A Journey of quality of Living", subscription price $12 per year. Contact the Coalition at 1010 Wayne Avenue, Silver springs, MD 20910, **1-301-650-8868**

National Comprehensive Cancer Network (NCCN) is an alliance of 15 of the nation's leading cancer centers. The NCCN, formed to create cancer-management strategies for large employers and third-party payers, is working to integrate the experience of the member cancer centers to guarantee the delivery of high-quality and cost-effective services to cancer patients. By accessing this web home page, you will have access to information on the 15 cancer centers in the alliance, including:

> **Johns Hopkins Oncology Center**
> **Fred Hutchinson Cancer Research Center**
> **Memorial Sloane-Kettering Cancer Center**
> **Dana Farber Cancer Institute**

On-line address:
http://www.cancer.med.umich.edu:80/NCCN/NCCN.html

NCI CancerFax Service combines the use of a computer and a facsimile (fax) machine to create a service enabling users to receive current cancer information with a fax machine. To use, call the CancerFax computer **(1-301-402-5874)** from the telephone on your fax machine. A voice at CancerFax will ask you to select English or Spanish and then instruct you on how to acquire the CancerFax Contents lists, which provide listings of the available information and the six-digit code numbers necessary to access

the data. After you obtain and review the list, call CancerFax again and the voice will guide you through the necessary steps to select and receive faxed printouts of your selections. The prerecorded voice informs users of the page length of the selections and when it was last updated. CancerFax is available 7 days a week, 24 hours a day, with no fee for the service. The only cost is the cost of the telephone call to the CancerFax computer in Bethesda, Maryland.
CancerFax Computer: 1-301-402-5874

National Bone Marrow Transplant Link (BMT Link) promotes support for transplant patients. 29209 Northwestern Hwy., #624, Southfield, MI 48034, **1-800-LINK-BMT (phone & fax)**

National Brain Tumor Foundation raises funds for research, connects patients for support, offers a national listing of support groups, and a national newsletter. 785 Market St. #1600, San Francisco, CA 94102, **1-800-934-CURE, 1-415-284-0208, fax: 1-415-284-0209.**

National Breast Cancer Coalition are advocacy groups having more than 300 member organizations and thousands of individuals working to find a cure for breast cancer through the National Action Network. 1707 L Street NW, #1060, Washington, D.C. 20036, **1-202-296-7477, fax: 1-202-265-6854**

National Health Information Center at **1-800-336-4797** is a health information referral service which puts health professionals and consumers/patients in touch with those organizations that can provide answers.

Where to Get Cancer Information and Assistance

NHIC's Internet address is:
http://nhic-nt.health.org
Email: nhicinfo@health.org

National Hospice Organization (NHO) offers information and referrals about hospice services. 1901 N. Moore St. #901, Arlington, VA 22209, **1-800-658-8898, fax: 1-703-525-5762**

National Kidney Cancer Association works to increase survival and improve care through information, sponsors research and acts as a patient advocate. 1234 Sherman Avenue, #203, Evanston, IL 60202-1375, **1-847-332-1051, fax: 1-847-332-2978, BBS: 1-847-332-1052**

National Marrow Donor Program is a computerized, congressionally funded network that maintains a data base of available tissue-typed marrow donor volunteers. 3433 Broadway Street, NE., #500, Minneapolis, MN 55413, **1-800-MARROW-2, fax: 1-612-627-5818**

National Marrow Donor Program Office of Patient Advocacy provides information that assists patients in: choosing a transplant center, working with insurance companies and employer benefits representatives to obtain or improve coverage for BMTs, locating alternative funding for transplantation; the office also monitors the donor search process to ensure that patients progress through the search in a timely manner, conducts personalized searches of current medical literature for patients, maintains a resource library on patient services and support groups, explains bone marrow transplantation, and assists referring physicians in performing unrelated

marrow donor searches. The National Marrow Donor Program maintains a registry of volunteers willing to donate marrow. Call **1-800-526-7809 or 612-627-5842** or contact at 3433 Broadway Street, NE, Suite 500, Minneapolis, MN 55413

National Second Surgical Opinion Hotline, **1-800-492-6833**, for assistance in locating a specialist in your area

The Oley Foundation offers support for home parenteral and/or enteral nutrition therapy patients, consumers, and families through publishing a newsletter, meetings, support activities. 214 Hun Memorial, Albany Medical Center A-23, Albany, NY. 12208, **1-800-776-OLEY**, fax: **1-518-262-5528**. Web address:
http://www.wizvax.net/oleyfdn

OncoLink is an information database covering all aspects of the cancer experience and is used by both the medical community and the general public. Accessing OncoLink puts you in contact with a huge number of resources, therefore adding to your resource file. Contact OncoLink via on-line at:
http://cancer.med.upenn.edu/
or voice telephone: **1-215-662-3084**

R.A. Bloch Cancer Foundation, Inc. assists patients get the best treatment through educational materials, peer counseling, medical second opinions, and support groups. The Cancer Hotline, 4410 Main Street, Kansas City, MO. 64111, **1-816-932-8453, fax: 1-816-931-7486.**

SHARE is an organization providing help for women with breast or ovarian cancer. They have many services and should be contacted for information and assistance. SHARE offers hotlines in English, Spanish and Chinese. They can be reached at: 1501 Broadway, Suite 1720, New York, N.Y. 10036

Support for People with Oral and Head and Neck Cancer, Inc. (SPOHNC) is a program of self help and support addressing emotional, psychological and humanistic needs of cancer patients. They publish a newsletter designed to increase awareness of head and neck cancer issues.
P.O. Box 53, Locust Valley, NY. 11560-0053, **1-516-759-5333 (phone & fax)**,
E-mail: spohnc@netcom.com

Susan G. Komen Breast Cancer Foundation is a national volunteer organization working to advance research for a cure. Hotline available. 5005 LBJ Freeway, #370, Dallas, TX 75244, **1-800-462-9273, fax: 1-214-450-1710**

The Wellness Community provides free psychosocial support to patients as an addition to conventional treatments. There are 16 facilities nationally.
2716 Ocean Park Blvd., #1040, Santa Monica, CA 90405-5211, **1-310-314-2555, fax: 1-310-314-7586**

United Ostomy Association, Inc. is an national association of chapters focusing on the rehabilitation of ostomy patients. 36 Executive Park, #120, Irvine, CA 92714, **1-800-826-0826, 1-714-660-8624, fax: 1-714-660-9262**

Y-Me Breast Cancer Organization is a National Breast Cancer Organization offering counseling, educational programs, and self-help meetings for patients and families. 212 W. Van Buren, 4th Fl., Chicago, IL 60617, **1-800-986-8228 (24-hour hotline), fax: 312/986-0020**

Your Daily Health is an information website service of The New York Times Information Services Group featuring timely, in-depth articles on health news topics. You can access the latest news on health issues, select specific health topics, and search for articles by keyword. Access the site at: http://www.yourhealthdaily.com/

Where to Get Cancer Information and Assistance

Web Service Engines

These Engines are designed to give you the ability to search the entire web for any topic. These sites index the entire web, covering all subjects, so you will access a lot of documents that contain your "search terms" but have nothing whatsoever to do with what you are actually looking for. Searching via these engines takes time and practice, and can result in some wasted "hits", but considering the immense amount of information and power available through these search engines, they are still an extremely valuable means of accessing information on cancer. Depending on who your net server is, you will have access to engines such as Yahoo, Alta Vista, HotBot, MetaCrawler, SavvySearch, Lycos, Excite and InfoSeek. Initiating a search just one of these web service engines will link you to so many resources that your Bookmark file will be filled in no time! A little practice will teach you which service engine is best for your needs, and you will be amazed at how quickly the on-line hours start to accumulate.

Internet News Groups

alt.support.cancer - technical and emotional support

sci.med.diseases.cancer - technical information and discussion

sci.med - general discussion of medicine

Online Library Catalogs

You can use online library catalogs to conduct a search for books on cancer and cancer-related issued. Many university libraries, and increasing numbers of local libraries maintain these catalogs. You can also conduct a search through Paperchase on Compuserve.

Audio Tapes

Books on Tape by Dr. Bernie S. Siegel, M.D.:
    <u>Love, Medicine & Miracles</u> (2-tape set)
    <u>Peace, Love, & Healing</u> (2-tape set)
    <u>How to Live Between Office Visits</u> (2-tape set)

Meditation Tapes by Bernie S. Siegel, M.D.:
    <u>Guided Imagery & Meditation</u>
    <u>Healing Meditations</u>
    <u>Meditations for Everyday Living</u>
    <u>Getting Ready: Meditations for Surgery, Chemo & Radiation</u>
    <u>Meditations for Peace of Mind</u>
    <u>Meditations for Finding the Key to Good Health</u>
    <u>Meditations for Enhancing Your Immune System</u>

Lecture Tapes by Bernie S. Siegel, M.D.:
    <u>Humor and Healing</u>
    <u>More Love, Medicine & Miracles</u>
    <u>Life, Hope & Healing: Prescriptions from the Heart</u> (6-tape set)

Note: The above tapes are available from ECAP, 1-800-700-8869 (Fax: 1-203-343-5950 or 5956)

Also:
    <u>Surgery</u>, Belleruth Naparstek
    <u>Chemotherapy, Depression, General Wellness, Surgery I&II</u>, Belleruth Naparstek

Note: Order from Image Paths, Inc., P.O. Box 5714, Cleveland, OH 44101, 1-800-800-8661

Appendix / CONTINUED

Alternative Therapies

We do not endorse or recommend any of the following; it is up to you to research and define their viability.

American Holistic Medicine Association provides a national directory of holistic physicians, the fee is currently $8. The address is: 4101 Lake Boone Trail, #201, Raleigh, N.C. 27607, **1-919-787-5181**

Cancer Control Society is a non-profit educational, charitable and scientific society supported by contributions and memberships. It offers information on alternative cancer treatments. Contact at 2043 North Berendo Street, Los Angeles, CA 90027, **1-213-663-7801**. **A fee is charged for mailed materials.

Health Quarters is a ministry focusing on the detoxification of the body and mind. Founded by Ann Frahm, author of Cancer Battle Plan, HealthQuarters offers an eleven-day retreat program. Additional books written by Ann are available along with videotape on how she survived breast cancer. P.O. Box 62130, Colorado Springs, CO. 80962, **1-719-593-8694**

Foundation for Advancement in Cancer Therapy at P.O. Box 1242, Old Chelsea Station, New York, N.Y., **1-212-741-2790**

Office of Alternative Medicine, National Institute of Health, 9000 Rockville Pike, Bldg. 31, Rm 513-38, Bethesda, MD. 20892, **1-800-531-1794** Call for information.

World Research Foundation is a worldwide organization offering reports on traditional and holistic medicine, quarterly newsletter and catalog of books and tapes. World Research Building, 41 Bell Rock Plaza, Ste. C, Sedona, AZ 86351, **1- 520-284-3300**

Travel Assistance

Air Care Alliance:
http://www.angelflightfla.org/aircareall.org/acahome.html
Telephone: **1-800- 296-1217**

Corporate Angels Network:
http://www.mach2media.com/can
Telephone: **1-914- 328-1313**

NPATH: the National Patient Air Transport Hotline: **1-800-296-2917**

Air Life Line: 1-800-446-1231

Angel flight: 1-800-296-1217
(c/o Air Care Alliance)

Air-Evac International, Inc.:
email: AirEvacInt@AOL.com
1-800-982-5806
or write: Air Evac International Inc., 21893 Skywest Drive, Hayward, CA 94541

Other:

For hair loss:

Look of Love International,
1913 Route 27, Edison, NJ 08817
(908) 572-3033. Wigs, head coverings.

For hair loss and mastectomy:

Hats with Heart, Inc.
10271 South 1300 East, Suite 166,
Sandy, Utah 84094.
For the nearest retailer or to order a catalog,
call **1-(800) 708-0066**. Wigs, hats, mastectomy apparel.

For dealing with treatment side effects:

Look Good - Feel Better, 1-800-395-LOOK
A program developed by the Cosmetic,
Toiletry and Fragrance Association, the
National Cosmetology Association and the
American Cancer Society and designed to
help patients take care of their hair, skin,
nails, and appearance.

NEUE Medical Products,
711 South Main Street, Burbank, CA 91506
(818) 563-4869 or (800) 832-8311 Offers
ALRA Oncology Care Products and NEUE
Antibacterial Products, including lotions,
shampoo, aloe vera gel, etc.

For information on insurance-covered standard treatment and clinical trials:

The Association of Community Cancer
Centers: (301) 984-9496 11600 Nebel St.,
Suite 201, Rockville, MD 20852 **Fax: 301-
770-1949**

Additional Resources

The Bone Marrow Transplant Special
Interest Group, 1996 Bone Marrow
"Transplant Nursing Resource Directory",
Oncology Nursing Press, Inc., Pittsburgh,
PA 15220-2749 1996.

Note: This book is published by the
ONS for use by oncology nurses. The directory
includes information on BMT programs at a
limited number of centers, and is not intended
as a comprehensive list of available programs.
Patients are encouraged to seek the advice of
their healthcare providers before making any
decisions about treatment or treatment facilities.
The ONS is located at 501 Holiday Drive,
Pittsburgh, PA 15220-2749, **1-412-921-7373**.

National Marrow Donor Program,
"Transplant Center Access Directory",
NMDP Office of Patient Advocacy,
Minneapolis, MN 55413

CANCER CENTERS

The institutions listed have been recognized as Cancer Centers by the National Cancer Institute. These centers have been rigorously reviewed by the National Cancer Advisory Board. They receive financial support from the National Cancer Institute, the American Cancer Society, and many other sources.

ALABAMA
University of Alabama at Birmingham*
Comprehensive Cancer Center
(205) 934-5077

ARIZONA
University of Arizona*
Arizona Cancer Center
(602) 626-6044

CALIFORNIA
The Kenneth Norris, Jr. Comprehensive
Cancer Center*
University of Southern California
(213) 740-2311

Jonsson Comprehensive Cancer Center*
University of California at Los angeles
(310) 825-5268

LaJolla Cancer Research Foundation
(619) 455-6480

University of California at San Diego
Cancer Center
(619) 543-3325

City of Hope Beckman Research Institute
(818) 359-8111

Armand Hammer Ctr. for Cancer Biology
Salk Institute
(619) 453-4100

COLORADO
University of Colorado Cancer Center
Univ. of Colorado Health Sciences Center
(303) 270-3007

CONNECTICUT
Yale University*
Comprehensive Cancer Center
(203) 785-4095

DISTRICT OF COLUMBIA
Lombardi Cancer Research Center*
Georgetown University Medical Center
(202) 687-2110

FLORIDA
Sylvester Comprehensive Cancer Center*
University of Miami Medical School
(305) 548-4918

ILLINOIS
University of Chicago
Cancer Research Center
(312) 702-6180

Lurie Cancer Center
Northwestern University
(312) 908-5250

INDIANA
Purdue University Cancer Center
(317) 494-9129

MAINE
The Jackson Laboratory
(207) 288-3371

MARYLAND
The Johns Hopkins Oncology Center*
(410) 955-8822

MASSACHUSETTS
Dana-FarberCancer Institute*
(617) 632-2155

Massachusetts Institute of Technology
Center for Cancer Research
(617) 253-6422

MICHIGAN
Meyer L. Prentis Comprehensive Cancer Center
Wayne State University
(313 745-8870

University of Michigan Comprehensive
Cancer Center*
(313) 936-2516

MINNESOTA
Mayo Clinic Comprehensive Cancer Center*
(507) 284-3413

NEBRASKA
Eppley Institute
University of Nebraska Medical Center
(402) 559-4238

NEW HAMPSHIRE
Norris Cotton Cancer Center*
Dartmouth-Hitchcock Medical Center
(603) 650-4141

NEW YORK
Cold Spring Harbor Laboratory
(516) 367-8383

Memorial Sloan-Kettering Cancer Center*
(212) 639-6561

Roswell Park Cancer Institute*
(716) 845-5770

Albert Einstein College of Medicine Cancer Research
Center
(718) 430-2302

Columbia-Presbyterian Cancer Center
Columbia University
(212) 305-6921

Kaplan Comprehensive Cancer Center*
New York University Medical Center
(212) 263-5349

University of Rochester Cancer Center
(716) 275-4911

American Health Foundation
(212) 953-1900

NORTH CAROLINA
Duke University Comprehensive Cancer Center*
(919) 684-3377

Lineberger Comprehensive Cancer Center*
University of North Carolina
(919) 966-3036

Wake Forest University*
Comprehensive Cancer Center
(910) 716-4464

OHIO
Ohio State University*
Comprehensive Cancer Center
Arthur G. James Cancer Hospital
(614) 293-4878

Case Western Reserve University
Cancer Research Center
(216) 368-1177

PENNSYLVANIA
Fox Chase Cancer Center*
(215) 728-2781

University of Pennsylvania Cancer Center*
(215) 662-6334
Wistar Institute Cancer Center
(215) 898-3926

Fels Institute
Temple University School of Medicine
(215) 707-4307

Pittsburgh Cancer Institute*
University of Pittsburgh
(412) 647-2072

TENNESSEE
Drew-Meharry-Morehouse
Consortium Cancer Center
(615) 327-6315

St. Jude Childrenís Research Hospital
(901) 495-3301

TEXAS
M.D. Anderson Cancer Center*
University of Texas
(713) 792-7500

San Antonio Cancer Institute
(210) 677-3850

UTAH
Huntsman Cancer Institute
University of Utah Health Sciences Center
(801) 581-4048

VERMONT
Vermont Regional Cancer Center*
University of Vermont
(802) 656-4414

VIRGINIA
Massey Cancer Center
Medical College of Virginia/VCU
(804) 828-0450

University of Virginia Cancer Center
(804) 924-9333

WASHINGTON
Fred Hutchinson Cancer Research Center*
(206) 667-4302

WISCONSIN
Comprehensive Cancer Center*
University of Wisconsin
(608) 263-8610

McArdle Laboratory for Cancer Research
University of Wisconsin Medical School
(608) 262-2177

*Indicates Comprehensive Cancer Center.
Reprinted by Permission of the American Cancer Society, Cancer
Facts and Figures, 1996

CHARTERED DIVISIONS
OF THE AMERICAN CANCER SOCIETY

Alabama Division, Inc.
504 Brookwood Boulevard
Homewood, Alabama 35209
(205) 879-2242

Alaska Division, Inc.
1057 West Fireweed Lane, Suite 204
Anchorage, Alaska 99503
(907) 277-8696

Arizona Division, Inc.
2929 East Thomas Road
Phoenix, Arizona 85016
(602) 224-0524

Arkansas Division, Inc.
901 North University
Little Rock, Arkansas 72207
(501)893-7900

California Division, Inc.
1710 Webster Street
Oakland, California 94604
(510)893-7900

Colorado Division, Inc.
2255 South Oneida
Denver, Colorado 80224
(303) 758-2030

Connecticcut Division, Inc.
Barnes Park South
14 Village Lane
Wallingford, Connecticut 06492
(203) 265-7161

Delaware Division, Inc.
92 Read's Way, Suite 205
New Castle, Delaware 19720
(302) 324-4227

District of Columbia Division, Inc.
1875 Connecticut Avenue, NW
Suite 730
Washington, DC 20009
(202) 483-2600

Florida Division, Inc.
3709 West Jetton Avenue
Tampa, Florida 33629-5146
(813) 253-0541

Georgia Division, Inc.
2200 Lake Blvd.
Atlanta, Georgia 30319
(404) 816-7800

Hawaii Pacific Division, Inc.
Community Services Center Bldg.
200 North Vineyard Blvd.,Suite 100-A
Honolulu, Hawaii 96817
(808) 531-1662

Idaho Division, Inc.
2676 Vista Avenue
Boise, Idaho 83705-0386
(208) 343-4609

Illinois Division, Inc.
77 East Monroe
Chicago, Illinois 60603-5795
(312) 641-6150

Indina Division, Inc.
8730 Commerce Park Place
Indianapolis, Indiana 46268
(317) 872-4432

Iowa Division, Inc.
8364 Hickman Road, Suite D
Des Moines, Iowa 50325
(515) 253-0147

Kansas Division, Inc.
1315 SW Arrowhead Road
Topeka, Kansas 666604
(913) 273-4114

Kentucky Division, Inc.
701 West Muhammad Ali Blvd.
Louisville, Kentucky 40201-1807
(502) 584-6782

Louisiana Division, Inc. 2200
Veterans' Memorial Blvd., Suite 214
Kenner, Louisiana 70062
(504) 469-0021

Maine Division, Inc.
52 Federal Street
Brunswick, Maine 04011
(207) 729-3339

Maryland Division, Inc.
8219 Town Center Drive
Baltimore, Maryland 21236-0026
(410) 931-6850

Massachusetts Division, Inc.
30 Speen Street
Framingham, Massachusetts 01701
(508) 270-4600

Michigan Divsion, Inc.
1205 East Saginaw Street
Lansing, Michigan 48906
(612) 925-2772

Mississippi Division, Inc.
1380 Livingston Lane
Lakeover Office Park
Jackson, Mississippi 39213
(601) 362-8874

Missouri Division, Inc.
3322 American Avenue
Jefferson City, Missouri 65102
(314) 893-4800

Montana Division, Inc.
17 North 26th Street
Billings, Montana 59101
(406) 2522-7111

Nebraska Division, Inc.
8502 West Center Road
Omaha, Nebraska 68124-5255
(402) 393-5800

Nevada Division, Inc.
1325 East Harmon
Las Vegas, Nevada 89119
(702) 798-6857

New Hampshire Division, Inc.
Gail Singer Memorial Bldg.
360 Route 101, Unit 501
Bedford, New Hampshire 03110-5032
(603) 472-8899

New Jersey Division, Inc.
2600 US Highway 1
North Brunswick, New Jersey 08902-0803
(908) 297-8000

New Mexico Division, Inc.
5800 Lomas Blvd., NE
Albuquerque, New Mexico 87110
(505) 260-2105

New York State Division, Inc.
6725 Lyons Street
East Syracuse, New York 13057
(315) 437-7025

Long Island Division, Inc.
75 Davids Drive
Hauppauge, New York 13057
(516) 436-7070

New York City Division, Inc.
19 West 56th Street
New York, New York 10019
(212) 586-8700

Queens Division, Inc.
112025 Queens Boulevard
Forest Hils, New York 11375
(718) 263-2224

Westchester Division, Inc.
30 Glenn Street
White Plains, New York 10603
(914) 949-4800

North Carolina Division, Inc.
11 South Boylan Avenue, Suite 221
Raleigh, North Carolina 27603
(919) 834-8463

North Dakota Division, Inc.
123 Roberts Street
Fargo, North Dakota 58102
(701) 232-1385

Ohio Division, Inc.
5555 Frantz road
Dublin, Ohio 43017
(614) 889-9565

Oklahoma Division, Inc.
4323 63rd, Suite 110
Oklahoma City, Oklahoma 73116
(405) 842-9888

Oregon Division, Inc.
0330 SW Curry
Portland, Oregon 97201
(503) 295-6422

Pennsylvania Division, Inc.
Route 422 & Sipe Avenue
Hershey, Pennsylvania 17033-0897
(717) 533-6144

Philadelphia Division, Inc.
1626 Locust Street
Philadelphia, Pennsylvania 19103
(215) 985-5400

Puerto Rico Division, Inc.
Calle Alverio #577
Esquina Sargento Medina
Hato Rey, Puerto Rico 00918
(809) 764-2295

Rhode Island Division, Inc.
400 Main Street
Pawtucket, Rhode Island 02860
(401) 722-8480

South Carolina Division, Inc.
128 Stonemark Lane
Westpark Plaza
Columbia, South Carolina 29210-3855
(803) 750-1693

South Dakota Division, Inc.
4101 S. Carnegie Place
Sioux Falls, South Dakota 57106-2322
(803) 750-1693

Tennessee Division, Inc.
1315 Eighth Avenue, South
Nashville, Tennessee 37203
(615) 255-1227

Texas Division, Inc.
2433 Ridgepoint Drive
Austin, Texas 78754
(512) 928-2262

Utah Division, Inc.
941 East 3300 South
Salt Lake City, Utah 84106
(801) 483-1500

Vermont Division, Inc.
13 Loomis Street, Drawer C
Montpelier, Vermont 05602

Virginia Division, Inc.
4240 Park Place Court
Glen Allen, Virginia 23060
(804) 527-3700

Washington Division, Inc.
2120 Sirst Avenue North
Seattle, Washington 98109-114-
(206) 283-1152

West Virginia Division, Inc.
2428 Kanawha Boulevard East
Charleston, West Virginia 25311
(304) 344-3611

Wisconsin Division, Inc.
N19 W24350 Riverwood Drive
Waukesha, Wisconsin 53188
(414) 523-5500

Wyoming Division, Inc.
4202 Ridge Road
Cheyenne, Wyoming 82001
(307) 638-3331

*Reprinted by permission of
the American Cancer Society*

Glossary of Medical Terms

Note: This glossary contains a list of medical terms that you may hear during the treatment of your cancer. Some of these words are used in the text of this book, but most are not. The purpose of this glossary is to give you a simple, understandable definition of the many words associated with cancer diagnosis and treatment. Never let a medical person use a word in discussing your condition and treatment that you do not understand without requesting an explanation of the terminology.

Ablative therapy - Surgical removal of a body part, or the destruction of its function.

Access device - A tube (catheter), placed into the chest, used to give chemotherapy, antibiotics and blood fluids. Also used to obtain blood samples.

Acini - The sac - like part of the milk - producing glands in the breast, also called lobules.

Acute - A sudden onset of symptoms or diseases.

Adenocinoma - Cancer that starts in the glands.

Adenoma - A benign growth that may or may not transform to cancer.

Adjuvant therapy - Additional treatment to increase the effectiveness of primary treatment, as in chemotherapy or radiation following surgery.

Adrenal gland - A gland near the kidney that produces adrenaline, cortisone, androgen, progestin, and possibly estrogen.

Advanced cancer - A stage of cancer in which the disease has spread from the primary site to other parts of the body.

Alopecia - Hair loss.

Analgesic - A drug that relieves pain. Aspirin is an analgesic.

Androgen - A male sex hormone. It can be used to treat recurrence of breast cancer as it will block the activity of estrogen which feeds some cancers.

Anemia - A condition caused by a decrease in the number of red blood cells. Symptoms included are tiredness, shortness of breath, and weakness.

Anesthesia - The loss of sensation as a result of drugs or gases.

Antibiotics - Chemical substances, produced by living organisms or synthesized in laboratories, for the purpose of killing other organisms that cause disease.

Antibodies - Proteins that are made as a response to the body recognizing a foreign substance.

Antidepressant - A medication to help relieve depression. Also used to help control tingling or burning from damaged nerves.

Antiemetics - Medications used to prevent or control nausea and vomiting.

Antiestrogen - A substance that blocks the effects of estrogen on tumors.

Antigen - An invading foreign agent, such as a virus, that causes antibodies to form.

Antimetabolites - Substances that interfere with the body's metabolic processes. In treating cancer, antimetabolite drugs disrupt DNA production, thus preventing cell division and tumor growth.

Antiseptic - A substance that stops or inhibits the growth of bacteria.

Areola - The dark area of flesh that encircles the nipple of the breast.

Artery - A large blood vessel carrying blood from the heart to other parts of the body.

Aspiration - The process of removing fluid from a specific area.

Asymptomatic - Without noticeable signs or symptoms of disease.

Attending Physician - doctor who has primary responsibility for patient care.

Axilla - The armpit.

Axillary dissection - A surgical procedure in which the lymph nodes in the armpit are remove and examined to determine if breast cancer has spread to those nodes.

Axillary node - Lymph node in the armpit.

Barium Enema - A milky substance (barium sulfate) is given rectally to allow x-rays to examine the lower intestines.

Barium swallow - The drinking of a milky substance (barium sulfate) to allow x-rays to examine the upper intestines.

Benign - The opposite of cancerous; does not spread to other parts of the body.

Bilateral - Affecting both sides of the body.

Biological response modifiers - A class of compounds, produced in the body, that boost the body's immune system to fight against cancer.

Biological therapy - The use of biologicals (substances produced by our own cells) or biological response modifiers (see previous definition) in the treatment of cancer.

Biopsy - The surgical removal for microscopic examination in order to determine whether cancer cells are present.

Blasts - Young, immature white blood cells.

Blood cells - Made in the bone marrow, they consist of red blood cells, white blood cells, and platelets.

Blood count - Measurement of the number of red cells, white cells, and platelets in a sample of blood.

Blood pressure - The pressure of blood on the walls of the arteries. The two measurements are *systolic*, the higher one which happens each time the heart pushes blood into the arteries, and the *diastolic*, or lower number which is the pressure at rest.

Blood vessel - Tube-like system of canals in the body to carry blood to and from body parts. The three main types are arteries, veins, and capillaries.

Bone marrow - The inner, spongy core of bone that produces blood cells.

Bone marrow transplant - A treatment wherein bone marrow is given back to a patient after they have received chemotherapy and radiation therapy. An Autologous BMT uses disease-free marrow harvested (removed) from the patient and either stored or given back to the patient following chemotherapy. An Allogeneic BMT uses marrow harvested from a donor that has been HLA matched to the patient. A Syngeneic BMT uses marrow donated by an identical twin.

Bone scan - An imaging method that gives important information about the growth and health of bones.

Bone survey (or Skeletal survey) - X-rays of the entire skeleton.

Brachytherapy - Internal radiation treatment achieved by implanting radioactive material directly into or near the tumor.

Brain scan - An imaging method used to find abnormalities in the brain.

BRCA1 - A gene located on the short arm of chromosome 17 which when mutated places a woman at greater risk of developing breast and/or ovarian cancer.

Breast augmentation - Surgery to increase the size of the breast.

Breast conservation therapy - Surgery to remove a breast cancer and a small amount of tissue around the cancer, without removing any other part of the breast. Also called a lumpectomy.

Breast implant - A manufactured sac that is filled with silicone gel or saline and surgically inserted to increase breast size or restore the appearance of a breast after mastectomy.

Bronchoscopy - A lighted tube is inserted through the mouth into the lungs for diagnostic purposes.

CA125II - A blood test used to mark proteins that may suggest tumor presence.

CEA - (Carcinoembryonic Agent) - A blood tumor test used to mark proteins that may suggest tumor presence.

Calcifications - Hardening of an organic substance by deposit of calcium salts within it. In the breast, these are signs of change that may be monitored by additional, periodic mammography, or by immediate or delay biopsy.

Cancer - A disease in which malignant cells grow out of control. Includes over 100 diseases.

Carcinogen - A substance or agent that is known to cause cancer.

Carcinoma - Cancer that begins in the tissues that line or cover an organ.

Catheter - A thin, plastic tube; when placed in a vein, it provides a pathway for drugs, nutrients, or blood products, and for the removal of blood samples.

CAT Scan - A test using x-rays to view organs and inside areas of the body.

Cauterization - The use of heat to destroy abnormal cells.

Cervix - The lower, narrow end of the uterus.

Chemotherapy - A treatment which destroys cancer cells with drugs.

Chronic - Persisting over a long period of time; chronic diseases progress slowly, are continuous or recurrent over long periods of time.

Clinical trial - The systematic investigation (study) of the effects of materials or methods, according to a formal study plan. Each study is designed to answer scientific questions and to find better ways to treat patients.

Colonoscopy - A test using a flexible, lighted tube inserted rectally to inspect the colon or large bowel.

Colony-stimulating factors - Substances that cause the body to produce new blood cells.

Colposcope - A magnifying instrument used to examine the vagina and cervix.

Combination chemotherapy - The use of more than one drug during cancer treatment.

Conization - The surgical removal of a cone-shaped piece of tissue from the cervix and cervical canal.

Contraindication - A treatment may not be helpful, and could be harmful.

Control group - In clinical studies, a group of patients which receives standard treatment, a treatment or intervention currently being used and considered to be of proved effectiveness on the basis of past studies. Results in patients receiving newly developed treatments may then be compared to the "control group".

Cryosurgery - Treatment with an instrument that freezes and destroys abnormal cells.

Cultures - Tests performed on body fluids, used to evaluate for the presence and type of infection. Tests take at least 24 hours to get first results and can take up to a full week to get final results.

Cytogenics - Testing that is performed on bone marrow samples and examines the chromosomes of cells. In leukemic patients, this test gives information about the type of leukemia that is present.

Cytotoxic - Any substance which is toxic to cells. Term is applied to drugs used to kill cancer cells.

Dietitian - A professional who plans diet programs for proper nutrition.

Differentiation - The process of cells maturing to become healthy adult cells.

Division - When a cell makes a copy of itself.

Double-blind - In a clinical trial, this is a characteristic of a controlled experiment in which neither the patient nor the attending physician knows whether the patient is on a particular drug or dosage. A special code identifies the treatment.

Drug resistant - The ability of cancer cells to resist the effects of a specific drug.

Dysphagia - Difficulty in swallowing.

Dysplasia - A non-cancerous condition that occurs when normal cells on the surface of the cervix are replaced by abnormal cells. Can be a precursor to cancer.

Dyspnea - Pain or difficulty in breathing, or shortness of breath.

Dysuria - Pain or difficulty in urination.

Effusion - Fluid build up in the body cavity, generally between two adjoining tissues.

Electron beam - A stream of Particles that produces high energy radiation for treating cancer.

Endometriosis - A benign condition in which endometrial tissue that looks like endometrial tissue grows in abnormal places in the abdomen or pelvis.

Endometrium - The inner lining of the uterus.

Endoscopy - A test using a probe to look inside the esophagus or stomach.

Erthrocyte - A red blood cell. It carries oxygen to body cells and carbon dioxide away from body cells.

Estrogen - A female hormone produced in the ovaries during the entire menstrual cycle.

Extended radical mastectomy - Surgical removal of the breast, skin, pectoral muscles, and all axillary and internal mammary lymph nodes on the same side.

Fats - One of the three main classes of food. They help the body use vitamins. They serve as sources of energy.

Fiber - Food substance found in plants. Fiber helps in the digestive process. The two types are soluble and insoluble.

Fine-Needle Aspirate - A needle is inserted into tissue to obtain a sample.

Free radicals - Naturally produced molecules which need to be neutralized or they can destroy DNA in cells. Over-stimulated by pollutants, they are thought to be the cause of some cancers.

Frozen section - Tissue removal quickly frozen and examined by a pathologist.

Gastrointestinal tracts - The digestive tract where food is processed; includes the stomach, liver, esophagus, small and large intestines and rectum.

Gene - A hereditary unit of DNA which tells the cells what and when to do something.

Gene Therapy - Specially manipulated targeted genes are inserted into a tumor to stimulate the immune system and kill off the tumor.

General anesthesia - Loss of consciousness as the result of the administration of drugs or gases.

Granulocytes - A type of white blood cell that kills bacteria.

Growth factors (hematopoietic) - Substances that stimulate blood cells to grow.

Gynecologic Oncology - Study and treatment of cancers related to the female reproduction organs.

Guided imagery - The use of mental images to promote healing; includes attitude and behavior changes.

Halsted radical mastectomy - Surgical removal of the breast, skin, both pectoral muscles, and all axillary lymph nodes on the same side.

Hematopoiesis - The process of blood cell growth.

Hematologist - A physician that specializes in the diseases and disorder of the blood.

Hickman catheter - Intravenous tubing that is surgically inserted into a large vein near the heart. The end of the catheter is tunneled under the skin and pulled out of an opening in the chest. Medications, fluids and blood products can be given through the catheter and blood can be withdrawn.

HMO (Health Maintenance Organization) - Type of medical coverage that dictates which doctors and medical facilities a patient can use.

Hormone - Chemical product of the endocrine glands of the body which has a specific effect on other organs when secreted into body fluids.

Hospice - Organization providing care given either at home or in the hospital to meet the needs of patients and family members during terminal illness stages.

HLA (human leukocyte antigen) - Proteins present on the surface of the body's cells, including bone marrow cells. Often referred to as transplantation antigens.

Hyperalimentation - Intravenous administration of solutions, generally nutrition based.

Hyperfractionated radiation - Division of the total dose of radiation into smaller doses that are given more than once per day.

Hyperplasia - An abnormal increase in the number of cells in a specific area.

Hysterectomy - An operation to remove the uterus.

Iliac crest - The hip bone area from which bone marrow samples are most commonly taken.

Ileostomy - An opening in the abdomen which allows stool to be collected into an external bag.

Imaging - Any method used to produce an image of internal body structures. Some methods used to detect cancer are x-rays, MRI, CAT scans, and ultrasonography.

Immune system - The system by which the body resists invasion by a foreign substance such as bacterial infection or a transplanted organ.

Immunocytochemistry - A method of detecting cancer in tissues, it involves using monoclonal antibodies to stain the tissues and cells before examination under a microscope.

Immunology - The study of how the body resists disease or invasion by foreign substances.

Immunosuppresion - A natural or induced stated in which the ability of the immune system to respond is decreased. Certain cancer therapies, including cytotoxic drugs, radiation and bone marrow transplant can cause immunosuppression.

Immunotherapy - Treatment that provokes or supports the body's immune system response to disease, such as cancer.

Indemnity Plan - Health care insurance that generally does not restrict choice of medical facilities or physicians.

Infiltrating ductal carcinoma - A cancer that starts in the milk ducts of the breast and then breaks through the duct wall where it invades the tissue of the breast. This cancer has the potential to metastasize.

Infiltration - Fluids that have leaked into tissues causing swelling.

Infusion pump - A pump that delivers fluids/medications into the bloodstream.

Intraclavicular nodes - Lymph nodes located beneath the collar bone (clavicle).

Interferon - A protein produced by cells, it helps regulate the body's defense system.

Interleukin-2 - A biological response modifier. It stimulates the growth of certain disease-fighting blood cells in the immune system. Also called IL-2.

Internal radiation therapy - See Brachytherapy

Internal mammary nodes - Lymph nodes beneath the breast bone one each side.

Intraductal papilloma - A benign tumor that begins in the ductal system of the breast.

Intramuscular - In a muscle.

Intraoperative - During surgery.

Intrathecal - Into the spinal fluid.

Intravenous (IV) - A method of supplying fluids and medications using a needle inserted into a vein.

Invasive - A term used to describe cancer that is able to invade and actively destroy surrounding healthy tissues.

Invasive lobular carcinoma - A cancer that arises in the lobules (milk producing glands) of the breast and then breaks through the lobule walls.

Investigational new drug - A drug allowed by the Food and Drug Administration (FDA) to be used in clinical trials, but not approved for commercial marketing.

Investigator - In clinical trials, the experienced clinical researcher who prepared a protocol or treatment plan and implements it with patients.

Isotope - Substance that gives off gamma, beta or alpha radiation.

Lactation - Production of milk in the breast.

Lattisimus dorse flap procedure - A method of breast reconstruction involving the use of the long flat muscle of the back by rotating it to the chest area.

Leukemia - Cancer of the organs that form the blood, such as lymph nodes and bone marrow.

Leukopenia - Decreased number of white blood cells in the blood.

Limited breast surgery - Also called lumpectomy, tylectomy, and segmental excision, it removes the breast cancer and a small amount of tissue around the cancer but preserves most of the breast. May be combined with axillary lymph node removal and radiation therapy.

Linear accelerator - A machine used in radiation therapy; it generates gamma rays and electron beams.

Lipid - A term for fat. The body breaks down lipids into fatty acids and burns them to get energy.

Local anesthesia - The loss of feeling or sensation in a specific area as the result of the administration of drugs or gases.

Local excision - The removal of a lesion or tumor that is confined to one area.

Lumpectomy - Surgery to remove a tumor and a small amount of surround normal tissue.

Lymph - Clear fluid that passes within the lymphatic system and contains cells known as lymphocytes; these cells fight infections.

Lymph nodes - Small bean-like nodes in the lymphatic system. The lymph system acts as a straining system for bacteria. It can also trap cancer cells. For certain types of cancer, the lymph nodes must be checked for cancer cells.

Lymphatic system - The tissue and organs that produce and store lymph. This includes bone marrow, spleen, thymus and lymph nodes.

Lymphedema - Swelling in the arm caused by excess fluid that collects after lymph nodes are removed by surgery or treated by radiation.

Lymphoma - Tumor made up of lymph node tissue.

Malignant - Virulent and dangerous; that which is likely to have a fatal termination. When used with the word tumor , means cancer.

Mammography - An x-ray of the breast.

Mammoplasty - Plastic surgery to reconstruct the breast or change the shape, size, or position of the breast.

Massage therapy - A general term for the manipulation and kneading of the muscles and soft tissue.

Mastectomy - Surgical removal of the breast.

Mastitis - Inflammation or infection of the breast.

Medical oncologist - A doctor who specializes in the use of chemotherapy to treat cancer.

Median time to elimination - The time it takes one half of a drug to leave the body.

Metabolism - The chemical process that sustains life. Food fuels the energy needed for the metabolic process.

Metastasis - The spreading of cancer to other areas of the body.

Metastatic cancer - Cancer which has spread from its original site to one or more additional body sites.

Micrometastases - The spread of cancer cells in groups so small that they can only be seen under a microscope.

Modified radical mastectomy - Surgical removal of the breast, skin, nipple, areola, and most of the axillary lymph nodes on the same side, leaving the chest muscles intact.

Monoclonal antibodies - Antibodies manufactured in the laboratory and designed to seek out specific foreign agents (antigens) on cancer cells as targets.

Multimodality therapy - The combined use of more than one method of treatment (ex.: surgery and chemotherapy).

Myometrium - The muscular outer layer of the uterus.

Needle aspiration - Removal of fluid from a cyst, or cells from a tumor, using a needle and syringe to pierce the skin, reach the cyst or tumor, and with suction, aspirate specimens for biopsy analysis.

Needle biopsy - See needle aspiration.

Needle localization - A biopsy procedure used when the lump is difficult to locate. Local anesthesia is injected to numb the area and a thin needle is inserted into the area

and guided via x-ray to the suspect area and held there with a tiny hood. The biopsy is taken via a hypodermic needle, as in needle aspiration.

Neoplasm - Any abnormal growth; neoplasms may be benign or malignant. Cancer is a malignant neoplasm.

Neuropathy - A disease of the nervous system; may be a side effect of certain cancer treatments.

Neutropenia - a decrease in the number of white blood cells.

Nodal status - A count of the number and location of lymph nodes in the armpit to which cancer has spread or has not spread. Used to forecast the risk of cancer recurrence and prognosis.

Node - Lymph glands.

Nodule - A small lump that can be located by touch.

Nuclear medicine scan - A method for viewing internal organs such as the brain, liver, or bone, in which small amounts of a radioactive substance (isotope) are injected into the bloodstream. The isotope is concentrated in organs that absorb it, where it can be traced and used to produce an image of the organ.

Nulliparous - A woman who has never given birth to a child.

Nurse practitioner - A nurse who has complete the registered nurse degree and then taken highly specialized training. Can work with the supervision of a physician; can take on additional duties in diagnosis and treatment of patients and in many states, may write prescriptions.

Oncogene - A type of gene found in the chromosomes of tumor cells.

Oncologist - A physician specially trained in the diagnosis and treatment of cancer.

Oncology nurse specialist (ONS) - A nurse who has taken highly specialized training in the field of cancer, after completion of the registered nurse degree. An ONS may mix and administer treatments, monitor patients, prescribe and provide aftercare, and teach and counsel patient and their families.

Oncology social worker - A person with a master's degree in social work who has specialized in the field of cancer.

Oophorectomy - Surgery to remove the ovaries.

Osteoporosis - Breakdown or disintegration of bone resulting in diminished and porous bone mass fractures.

PDQ - A computerized database supported by the NCI and available to physicians nationwide. It is geographically matrixed and offers the latest information on standard treatments and ongoing clinical trials for each type and stage of cancer.

Paget's disease of the nipple - A breast cancer that begins in the milk passages and involves the skin of the nipple and areola.

Palliative treatment - Therapy that relieves symptoms, but does not cure the disease.

Palpation - Using the hands to examine.

Partial mastectomy - Surgical removal of less than the whole breast, taking only the part of the breast in which the cancer occurs and margin of surrounding healthy tissue.

Pathologist - A physician who specializes in the identification of abnormalities and disease by examining body tissue and organs under a microscope.

Pathology - The study of disease.

PDQ - An NCI supported database listing the latest information on standard treatments and clinical trials.

Pectoral muscles - Muscles attached to the front of the chest wall and upper arms.

Permanent section - The preparation of tissue for microscopic examination.

Pituitary gland - The main endocrine gland. It produces hormones that control other glands and many body functions, especially growth.

Placebo - An inert, inactive substance (sometimes called a "sugar pill"); may be used in clinical trials for comparative studies.

Ploidy - A measure of the amount of DNA contained in a cell. Used in determining how cancerous a tumor's cells are.

Polyunsaturated Fats - Fat that comes from vegetables.

Port - A small plastic or metal container surgically placed under the skin and atached to a central venous catheter inside the body. Blood and fluids can enter or leave the body through the port.

Precancerous - See premalignant.

Predisposition - Susceptibility to a disease.

Premalignant - Abnormal changes in cells that may become cancerous.

Primary cancer - The site where cancer begins.

Progesterone - A female sex hormone released by the ovaries.

Progesterone receptor assay - A test that shows whether a breast cancer depends on progesterone for growth.

Prognosis - A prediction of the course of disease.

Prolactin - A hormone released by the pituitary gland that prompts lactation.

Prophylactic mastectomy - Surgical removal of the interior of one or both breast before any cancer is found for the purpose of preventing cancer.

Prosthesis - An artificial substitute for a missing part. (Plural: prostheses)

Protein - One of the three classes of food. They are made of amino acids, which are called the building blocks of life. Cells need protein to grow and heal themselves.

Protocol - A formalized outline or plan.

Quandrantectomy - A partial mastectomy in which the quarter of the breast that contains the tumor is removed.

Rad - Short for "radiation absorbed dose". It is a measurement of the amount of radiation absorbed by tissues.

Radiation oncologist - A doctor who specializes in using radiation to treat cancer.

Radioactive implant - A source of high-dose radiation placed temporarily into and around a cancer to kill the cancer cells.

Radioisotope - An isotope that is radioactive.

Radiologic technician - A health professional trained to properly position patients for x-rays, load film and take images, and develop and check the images for quality.

Radioimmunoscintigraphy (RIS) - A type of scan that seems to be more sensitive and accurate in predicting persistent or recurrent ovarian cancers that have no symptoms and no reactive tumor marker blood tests.

Radiologist - A physician who has received years of additional training to produce and read x-rays and other images (ultrasound, MRI, etc.) for the purpose of diagnosing abnormalities.

Radionuclide scanning - An examination that produces pictures of internal parts of the body; involves ingestion or injection of a small amount of radioactive material followed by examination by a scanner.

Radiosensitizers - Drugs being studied to try to boost the effect of radiation therapy.

Radiotherapy - Treatment with radiation to destroy cancer cells.

Randomized clinical trial - A study in which patients with similar traits, such as the extent of disease, are chosen or selected by chance to be placed in separate groups that are comparing different treatments.

Rectus abdominus flap procedure - Breast reconstruction in which tissue from the lower abdominal wall is used to create a breast.

Recurrence - Cancer that has re-occurred or reappeared after treatment.

Regression - The state of growing smaller or disappearing, used to describe the shrinkage or disappearance of cancer.

Relapse - Reappearance of cancer after a disease-free period.

Remission - A temporary or permanent stage or condition when cancer is not active and symptoms disappear. Although not synonymous with "cure", a nice word to hear nonetheless.

Risk factor - Something that increases a person's chance of developing a disease.

Risk/benefit ratio - The relation between the risks and benefits of a given treatment or procedure.

Sarcoma - A malignant tumor growing from connective tissues, such as cartilage, fat, muscle or bone.

Saturated fat - A type of fat that comes from animals.

Scan - A study using x-rays or radioactive isotopes to produce images of internal body organs.

Scintillation camera - A device used to enhance radiation and record the results for the diagnosis of cancer or other disorders.

Scirrhous cancer - Breast cancer with a hard, firm, fibrous texture.

Segmental mastectomy - See Partial mastectomy.

Shunt - A devise for passing blood from one area to another by means other than the usual channel.

Side effects - Problems that occur when treatment affects healthy cells. Ex.: fatigue, nausea, decreased blood cell counts, hair loss, mouth sores.

Simple mastectomy - Former term for Total mastectomy. See Total mastectomy.

Single blind - In clinical trials, the characteristic of a controlled experiment in which patients do not know which of several treatments they are receiving. The physicians are aware of the treatment the patient is receiving.

S-phase fractation (SPF) - The percentage of cells in a tumor that are in the Synthesis phase of dividing. Low SPF indicates a slow-growth tumor; high SPF indicates rapid tumor growth.

Staging - Methods used to establish the extent of a patient's disease.

Standard treatment - A treatment or other intervention currently being used and considered to be of proven effectiveness on the basis of past studies.

Stereotactic core needle biopsy - Needle biopsy in which computerized equipment is used to locate the suspect mass and guide the placement of the needle.

Stomatitis - Inflammation or ulcers of the lips, gums, tongue, palate, floor of the mouth, or other tissues in the mouth.

Study arm - In clinical trials, patients assigned to one part or segment of a study.

Subcutaneous injection - An injection of fluid into tissue under the skin.

Supraclavicular nodes - Lymph nodes above the collarbone (clavicle).

Systemic disease - Tumors that have spread to distant sites.

Systemic therapy - Treatment that reaches and affects cells throughout the body.

T-Cell - A white blood cell (lymphocyte) critical to the function of the immune system; fights foreign invaders.

Tissue - A group or layer of similar cells that perform a special function.

Total mastectomy - Surgical removal of the breast.

Toxins - Poisons produced by certain animals, plants, or bacteria.

TRAM flap (Transverse rectus abdominal muscle flap) - see Rectus abdominus flap procedure.

Treatment port or field - The place on the body at which the radiation beam is aimed.

Tumor - Tissue growth in which cells multiply uncontrollably. Also called neoplasm.

Tumor marker - A substance in the blood, such as a protein, that suggests that cancer may be present.

Tylectomy - see Lumpectomy.

Ultrasound - Imaging method using high-frequency sound waves to outline a part of the body.

Vital - Necessary to maintain life. Ex.: breathing.

X-rays - A form of radiation that can, at low levels, produce an image of cancer on film. At high levels it can destroy cancer cells.

Yoga - A range of exercise used to encourage well-being and the interaction of mind, body, and energy.

Suggested Readings

A New Prescription for Women's Health
Bernadine Healy, M.D.; Viking, 1995

Ageless Body, Timeless Mind
Deepak Chopra, M.D.; Harmony Books, 1993

Breast Cancer: The Complete Guide
Y. Hirshaut and P. Pressman; Bantam, 1993

Cancer Battle Plan
Anne E. Frahm with David Frahm, Pion Press, 1992

Cancervive: The Challenge of Life After Cancer
Susan Nessim and Judith Ellis; Houghton-Mifflin, l991

Coping with Chemotherapy
N. Bruning; The Dial Press, Rev. Ed. 1993

Dr. Susan Love's Breast Book
Susan Love; Addison-Wesley, 1990

Everyone's Guide to Cancer Therapy
Malin Dollinger, M.D., Ernest H. Rosenbaum, M.D., and
Greg Cable; Andrews and McMeel, 2nd Ed., 1994

Getting Well Again
Dr. O. Carl Simonton; Bantam Books

Gilda's Disease
Dr. Steven Piver with Gene Wilder; 1996

Healing Miracles
Dr. William A. McGarey, M.D.; St. Martin's, 1988

How to Live Between Office Visits (Audio Tapes)
Dr. Bernie S. Siegel, M.D.; Harper Collins, 1993

It's Always Something
Gilda Radner; Simon & Schuster, 1989

Love, Medicine & Miracles
Dr. Bernie S. Siegel, M.D.; Harper & Row. 1986

Mind as Healer, Mind as Slayer
Kenneth R. Pelletier; Delta, 1992

Minding The Body, Mending The Mind
Joan Borysenko, PH. D.; Addison-Wesley Publishing
Company, Inc., 1987

Natural Health, Natural Medicine,
Dr. Andrew Weil; Houghton Mifflin

Peace, Love & Healing
Dr. Bernie S. Siegel, M.D.; Harper & Row, 1989

Smart Medicine
Dr. Bruce Hensel; Berkley, 1989

Staying Well with Guided Imagery
Belleruth Naperstek; Warner, 1994

The Healing Journey
Dr. O. Carl Simonton; Bantam Books

The Ostomy Book: Living comfortably with
Colostomies, Ileostomies and Urostomies
Barbara Dorr; Mullen and Kerry McGin; Bull Publishing,
1992

The Power is Within You
Louise L. Hay; Hay House, 1991

The Road Back to Health: Coping with the Emotional
Side of Cancer, Neil A. Fiore; Bantam, 1984

You Can Heal Your Life
Louise L. Hay; Hay House, 1989

BIBLIOGRAPHY

A New Prescription for Women's Health, Bernadine Healy, M.D., Viking, 1995

1996 Bone Marrow Transplant Nursing Resource Directory, Oncology Nursing Society, 1996

Acute Myelogenous Leukemia; Leukemia Society of America, P-32 75M 7/94

Advanced Cancer; NIH Publication No. 93-856

Barnes and Noble Concise Medical Dictionary, Barnes & Noble Books, 1995

Beth Israel Patientís Guide to Breast Cancer/Treatment; http//www.wp.com/bicbs/gtreat.html

Breast Cancer Dictionary; American Cancer Society, No. 4675

Cancer Treatments Your Insurance Should Cover, The Association of Community Cancer Centers, 1991

CancerGuide: Specific Cancers, Steve Dunnís Cancer Information Page, Internet: Cancerguide.org; 1996

Chemotherapy and You, NIH Publication No. 94-1136

Choosing a BMT Center; BMT Newsletter, January 1994

Cleveland Clinic - Cancer Document; http://medhlp.netusa.net/ccf/howw2choz.htm

Colostomy: A Guide; American Cancer Society, No. 4703

Dealing with Outstanding Medical Bills, et al, OncoLink Team, Univ. of Penn. Cancer Center, 1996

Eat Better - Feel Better; American Cancer Society, Greater Hartford Chapter

Eating Hints for Cancer Patients; NIH Publication No. 94-2079

Facing Forward; NIH Publication No. 93-2424

Facts on Colorectal Cancer; American Cancer Society, No. 2004-LE

Facts on Testicular Cancer; American Cancer Society, No. 2645-L

Facts on Uterine Cancer; American Cancer Society, No. 2006-LE

Fighting Disease: The Complete Guide to Natural Immune Powers; Rodale Press, 1989. Out of print.

Fitting the Pieces Together, American Cancer Society, No.8601

The Healing Foods Cookbook; The Rodale Press, 1991

Hospice: A Special Kind of Caring; American Cancer Society, No. 4613

Ileostomy: A Guide; American Cancer Society, No. 4711

IMF - Nutritional and Dietary Management; Microsoft Interntet, Stacy Plotkin M.S, R.D., Cedars Inner Cleansing, Parker Publishing, 1992

Laughter Has Myriad Benefits; The New York Times Company, 1996

Living Wills and Other Advance Directives, http://mobar.org/brochure, 1996

Longevity, Longevity International, Ltd., March, 1995

Look Good, Feel Better; American Cancer Society, No. 4663.06

Love, Medicine & Miracles; Bernie Siegel, M.D., Harper & Row, Publishers, 1986

Minding the Body, Mending the Mind; Joan Borysenko, Ph.D., Addison-Wesley Publishing Company, Inc., 1987

MRI Patient Information; http://www.waterw.com/~Wstuff/mri.html#1

National Cancer Institute; web page, Patient Education: Adult - Microsoft Internet Explorer

New England Journal of Medicine, December Issue, Massachusetts Medical Society, 1989

Nuclear Medicine Bone Scans; http://www.bih.harvard.edu/radiolog Öucmed/nucmedSubdivsf/boneScans.html

Prescription for Nutritional Healing; James F. Balch, M.D., Phyllis A. Balch, C.N.C.. Avery Publishing Group, Inc., 1990

Preventing Cancer; The American College of Obstetricians and Gynecologists

Prevention and Treatment of Lymphedema; Microsoft Internet Explorer, Oncolink

Questions and Answers About the PLCO Cancer Screening Trial; CancerWEB, http://www.graylab.ac.uk/cancernet/600512.html

Radiation Therapy and You; American Cancer Society, No. 95-2227

Remedy; Sept/Oct 195, Making Time to Relax

Research Report: Bone Marrow Transplantation and Peripheral Blood Stem Cell Transplantation, NIH Publication No. 95-1179, revised 1994

Services for People with Cancer, People with Cancer, N.I.H.

Smart Medicine; Bruce Hensel, M.D., G.P. Putnam & Sons, 1989

Taking Time; NIH Publication No. 94-2059

The Trouble With HMOs, Ladies Home Journal; November 1996

Transplant Center Access Directory, The NMDP Office of Patient Advocacy, 1996

Understanding Chemotherapy, Leukemia Society of America, 1990

Urostomy: A Guide; American Cancer Society, No. 4709

What are Clinical Trials All About?; http://nysernet.org/bcic/nci/adult/clin.trials.92-2706/clin.trials.html

What Happens When You Eat, Electro-Medical Devices, Inc.

What you Need to Know About Bladder Cancer; NIH Publication No. 93-1559

What You Need to Know About Brain Tumors; NIH Publication No. 93-1558

What You Need to Know About Cancer; NIH Publication No. 94-1563

What You Need to Know About Cancer of the Bone; NIH Publication No. 93-1571

What You Need to Know About Cancer of the Cervix; NIH Publication No. 90-2047

What You Need to Know About Cancer of the Uterus; NIH Publication No. 93-1562

What You Need to Know About Hodgkinís Disease; NIH Publication No. 93-1555

What You Need to Know About Lung Cancer; NIH Publication No. 93-1553

What You Need to Know About Multiple Myeloma; NIH Publication No. 93-1575

What You Need to Know About Non-Hodgkinís Lymphomas; NIH Publication No. 93-1567

What You Need to Know About Ovarian Cancer; NIH Publication No. 94-1561

What You Need to Know About Prostate Cancer; NIH Publication No. 93-1576

What You Need to Know About Stomach Cancer; NIH Publication No. 94-1554

What You Need to Know About Testicular Cancer; NIH Publication No. 93-1565

ORDER FORM
A Copy For A Friend In Need

Our <u>correct</u> web address and e-mail:
Web: cancersos.com
e-mail: cancrsos@iag.net
(errors on order forms in back of book)

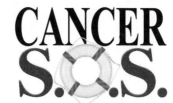

CANCER S.O.S.

Strategies Of Survival

A GUIDEBOOK FOR WOMEN WITH CANCER
by
Rose Welsh and Shirley Grandahl

1-800-818-8208

Fax or Mail:

_____
NAME

_____
STREET ADDRESS

_____
CITY   **STATE**   **ZIP CODE**   **COUNTRY**

❑ **CHECK**   ❑ **MASTERCARD**   ❑ **VISA**

CREDIT CARD # _____

NAME ON CARD _____ **EXPIRATION DATE** _____

I would like to order:

_____ **NUMBER OF BOOKS ORDERED @ $24.95 ea.** $_____.____

IN FLORIDA: ADD 7% SALES TAX $_____.____

SHIPPING & HANDLING: ADD $5.95 FIRST BOOK $_____.____

(ADD $3.00 Shipping & Handlingsecond book ordered) $_____.____
Call for rates on 3 or more books and special shipping

TOTAL PURCHASE $_____.____

Fax orders to: 407/330-3433
On-Line orders to: cancrsos.com
To order by mail: **Alba Publishing, Inc.**
P.O. Box 2918
Lake Mary, Florida 32795-2918

Please allow 7-10 days for delivery. 2 Day delivery available for additional fee.

Return Policy: Books may be returned within 2 weeks of delivery if unopened.

ORDER FORM
A Copy For A Friend In Need

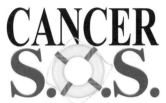

CANCER S.O.S.

Strategies Of Survival

A GUIDEBOOK FOR WOMEN WITH CANCER
by
Rose Welsh and Shirley Grandahl

Our <u>correct</u> web address and e-mail:
Web: cancersos.com
e-mail: cancrsos@iag.net
(errors on order forms in back of book)

1-800-818-8208

Fax or Mail:

_____

NAME

_____

STREET ADDRESS

_____

| CITY | STATE | ZIP CODE | COUNTRY |

❏ CHECK ❏ MASTERCARD ❏ VISA

CREDIT CARD # _____

NAME ON CARD _____ EXPIRATION DATE _____

I would like to order:

_____ **NUMBER OF BOOKS ORDERED @ $24.95 ea.** $_____.____

IN FLORIDA: ADD 7% SALES TAX $_____.____

SHIPPING & HANDLING: ADD $5.95 FIRST BOOK $_____.____

(ADD $3.00 Shipping & Handlingsecond book ordered) $_____.____
Call for rates on 3 or more books and special shipping

TOTAL PURCHASE $_____.____

Fax orders to: 407/330-3433
On-Line orders to: **cancrsos.com**
To order by mail: **Alba Publishing, Inc.**
                        P.O. Box 2918
                        Lake Mary, Florida 32795-2918

Please allow 7-10 days for delivery. 2 Day delivery available for additional fee.

Return Policy: Books may be returned within 2 weeks of delivery if unopened.